Interactive Music Therapy in
Child and Family Psychiatry

companion volume

Interactive Music Therapy – A Positive Approach
Music Therapy at a Child Development Centre
Amelia Oldfield
Foreword by Dr Fatima Janjua
ISBN 1 84310 309 5

of related interest

Pied Piper
Musical Activities to Develop Basic Skills
John Bean and Amelia Oldfield
ISBN 1 85302 994 7

Filling a Need While Making Some Noise
A Music Therapist's Guide to Pediatrics
Kathy Irvine Lorenzato
Foreword by Kay Roskam
ISBN 1 84310 819 4

**Multimodal Psychiatric Music Therapy for Adults,
Adolescents, and Children**
A Clinical Manual
Third Edition
Michael D. Cassity and Julia E. Cassity
ISBN 1 84310 831 3

Receptive Methods in Music Therapy
Techniques and Clinical Applications for Music Therapy Clinicians,
Educators and Students
Denise Grocke and Tony Wigram
ISBN 1 84310 413 X

Music Therapy – Intimate Notes
Mercédès Pavlicevic
ISBN 1 85302 692 1

Improvisation
Methods and Techniques for Music Therapy Clinicians,
Educators, and Students
Tony Wigram
Foreword by Professor Kenneth Bruscia
ISBN 1 84310 048 7

Songwriting
Methods, Techniques and Clinical Applications for Music Therapy Clinicians,
Educators and Students
Edited by Felicity Baker and Tony Wigram
Foreword by Even Ruud
ISBN 1 84310 356 7

Interactive Music Therapy in Child and Family Psychiatry

Clinical Practice, Research and Teaching

Amelia Oldfield

Foreword by Joanne Holmes

Jessica Kingsley Publishers
London and Philadelphia

First published in 2006
by Jessica Kingsley Publishers
116 Pentonville Road
London N1 9JB, UK
and
400 Market Street, Suite 400
Philadelphia, PA 19106, USA

www.jkp.com

Library of Congress Cataloging in Publication Data

Oldfield, Amelia.
Interactive music therapy in child and family psychiatry : clinical practice, research, and
teaching / Amelia Oldfield ; foreword by Joanne Holmes. -- 1st American pbk. ed.
    p. cm.
Includes bibliographical references and index.
ISBN-13: 978-1-84310-444-5 (pbk. : alk. paper)
ISBN-10: 1-84310-444-X (pbk. : alk. paper) 1. Music therapy for children. 2. Child
psychiatry. I. Title.
ML3920.O39 2006
616.89'16540083--dc22

2006023017

British Library Cataloguing in Publication Data
A CIP catalogue record for this book is available from the British Library

ISBN-13: 978 1 84310 444 5
ISBN-10: 1 84310 444 X

Printed and bound in Great Britain by
Athenaeum Press, Gateshead, Tyne and Wear

Contents

List of Tables

List of Figures

Foreword

Music therapists should come with a government health warning: *This therapist may seriously change the way you see the world!* In this regard, Amelia Oldfield would certainly be a high-risk therapist. In this delightfully straightforward and readable book, Amelia describes her interactive music therapy approach and how this is applied in the many varied aspects of her work. Her writing, like its author, is personal and approachable; accessible to both therapists and non-therapists alike.

I have worked with Amelia at the Croft Child and Family Unit since 1998. Until taking up my post in the unit my exposure to the creative therapies had been limited. Since then I have had the privilege of learning from Amelia and her music therapy colleagues the invaluable contribution that music therapy can make in an intensive child and adolescent mental health setting.

The Croft Unit is a residential mental health unit providing intensive assessment and treatment for children and families living in the East Anglian region of the UK. Most of the children attending the unit have severe and complex difficulties in multiple areas. These may include problems with emotion regulation and expression, learning difficulties, poor attention and impaired socio-communication skills. These children challenge both families and professionals by the breadth and variability of their difficulties.

During an admission it is vital that we see children and their families in a variety of settings so that we can identify areas of strength as well as difficulty. Over years I have noted that the children (and their parents) often display quite different aspects of this profile within the music therapy setting.

For very many children, music making is the highlight of their week, an opportunity to have fun and explore a different world. For children with speech and language problems it can be a rare chance to communicate through a non-verbal channel. For other children, as Amelia sensitively describes in this work, it can be the catalyst for rebuilding self-esteem or a damaged relationship.

Music therapists also bring their innovation and creative thinking to the rest of the multi-disciplinary team. My experience is that by sharing their enthusiasm for music making and relationship making with the wider team they can infect us all with hope for positive change for a child or family.

Not content with clinical work and training the next generation of music therapists, Amelia has also thrown herself into the rigours of academic research by producing groundbreaking work with direct clinical relevance. In this, as in all things, Amelia is generous in sharing her wealth of experience and insight.

This book provides the reader with a window into a unique music therapist's world. For the therapist it will provide a rich resource of clinical material and insight into Amelia's interactive work and the many different ways that music therapy can contribute to the assessment and treatment of children and families with complex mental health difficulties. For all of us this is an inspiring book that will provoke thought and innovation.

Dr Joanne Holmes BA, MRCPsych
Consultant Child and Adolescent Psychiatrist

Acknowledgements

Thank you to all the children and the families I have worked with, for providing me with the inspiration to write this book.

Thank you to all my colleagues who have helped, inspired and supported me over many years.

Thank you to Jo Holmes for writing the introduction. Thank you also for taking part in the research project with me and providing support and encouragement at all times.

Thank you to Emma Davies for allowing me to include her case studies in Chapter 3, for writing about the experience of individual supervision in Chapter 9, and generally for being an inspired, creative and supportive colleague for the past five years.

Thank you to Philippa Derrington, Susan Greenhalgh, Elinor Everitt, Kathryn Nall and Jo Tomlinson for your invaluable and moving contributions to Chapter 9.

Thank you to Christine Franke for many inspiring discussions and for writing about song stories with me.

Thank you to Malcolm Adams for continuous help with my research, over a period of 25 years.

Thank you to Claire Rawson for writing out the song.

Thank you to the children and families for allowing me to include their photographs.

Thank you to Joy Nudds and Melanie Piper for making stills from my music therapy training video.

Thank you to my husband, David, and my children Daniel, Paul, Laura and Claire, for letting me get on with my writing and being patient and encouraging.

A very special thank you to Phyllis Champion, for once again reading, re-reading and editing this book. You have continued to be positive and supportive, and have enabled the whole process of writing to be exciting and fulfilling. I look forward to working together again on future projects.

Introduction

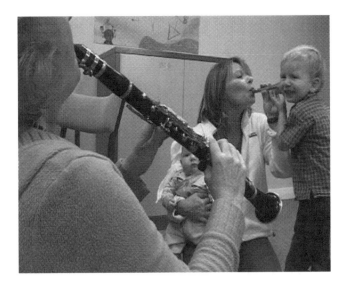

In my companion book (Oldfield 2006), I define 'interactive music therapy' and explain how this approach arose from clinical practice and research while working with pre-school children with autistic spectrum disorder and their parents. The work I shall be describing here also grew out of my clinical work. In addition I was influenced by the fact that the general role of the Croft children's unit, where I worked, gradually changed from being a treatment centre to becoming an assessment unit, and by the fact that an out-patient parenting project was run there for a number of years. Opportunities to develop music therapy approaches in specific clinical areas presented themselves.

Another factor was that my work and my approach in child and family psychiatry evolved, grew and defined itself because of my involvement with teaching music therapy students. In 1994, I jointly set up an MA music therapy training course at Anglia Ruskin University (previously named Anglia Polytechnic University) with my colleague Helen Odell Miller. Presenting clinical work to students, lecturing about theoretical aspects of my work and having to answer searching questions helped me to explain and understand my own work.

After a general introductory chapter, this book describes my interactive music therapy approach in a number of clinical areas within child and family psychiatry: music therapy diagnostic assessments, an open music therapy group, short-term individual treatment and work with families. I then describe a research investigation into music therapy diagnostic assessments. Finally, I reflect on my role as a music therapy supervisor and teacher.

Chapter 1

Characteristics of My Music Therapy Approach in Child and Family Psychiatry

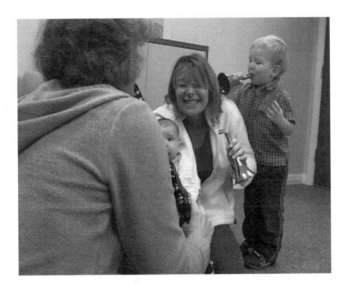

Introduction

This chapter first describes the Croft Unit for Child and Family Psychiatry and gives an outline of the history of music therapy at the unit. Because my music therapy approach has evolved from my clinical work I then include two vignettes. There then follows a description and definition of my approach and a reflection on how I have been influenced by other music therapists and by my own past and present experiences.

The Croft Unit for Child and Family Psychiatry

The Croft children's unit is a psychiatric assessment centre for children up to the age of 12 years and their families. There are usually no more than eight children attending at any one time. In the last couple of years the most common diagnoses of children seen at the unit have been attention deficit disorder (with or without hyperactivity), autistic spectrum disorders including autism and Asperger's syndrome, Gilles de la Tourette's syndrome, developmental delay, specific language disorders and conduct disorders. Although some families are admitted residentially, other children attend on a daily basis and regular meetings are arranged with the parents. Children are generally admitted only if their parents agree to work closely with staff on the unit. Assessments may last from two to six weeks. Occasionally, some children will attend for a longer specific piece of work that might last from 12 weeks to 6 months. During the day the children attend a unit school in the morning. In the afternoon they attend various groups, such as social skills, art and recreation groups which are run by unit staff.

Staff on the unit include psychiatrists, a family therapist, specialist nurses, a teacher, classroom assistants, health care assistants, clinical psychologists and music therapists. Social workers, health visitors and the teachers involved with the children outside the unit work closely with staff on the unit.

The strengths and difficulties of the children and the families admitted to the Croft are evaluated in various ways. The clinical psychologist carries out a number of psychological tests such as the Parenting Stress Index (PSI; Abidin 1995) as well as other cognitive or developmental tests on the children such as the Wechsler Intelligence Scale for Children (WISC). Sometimes special questionnaires are devised by the clinical psychologist for other members of staff on the unit to fill in, particularly when we are trying to observe and understand children's or families' difficulties that occur in unpredictable and erratic ways. Specially trained staff carry out Autistic Diagnostic Observation Schedule (ADOS) and Autistic Diagnostic Interview (ADI) tests (Dilavore *et al.* 1995; Lord *et al.* 1989). The teacher on the unit writes detailed reports not only on the academic strengths and weaknesses of the children but particularly on the children's abilities to learn and general behaviour in the classroom. Families will be interviewed, and observed in play sessions. In addition, staff assess the children and the families in less formal settings such as in the playground, at mealtimes and in the evenings, writing detailed notes in the families' files on a daily basis. In some cases, detailed physical records of children's weight and height, as well as bowel movements and sleeping patterns, are carefully monitored.

History of music therapy at the Croft

The part-time music therapy post at the Croft was first established in 1985. I took on the post in 1987. At that time the unit was mainly a treatment centre which admitted children for a minimum of six weeks but usually for three months to a year. Initially, my work involved mainly treating individual children, groups of children, families or groups of mothers and young children while liaising regularly with the team about the work that I was doing. Gradually, the unit has become a diagnostic centre, mainly only admitting children and families for four weeks, although occasionally one or two families or children will be admitted for treatment for several months. I have, therefore, had to radically rethink and change my ways of working, adapting previous music therapy treatment methods to short-term work (rarely more than four to six sessions) and to music therapy diagnostic assessments (two half-hour individual sessions).

Two vignettes

Damien

Damien was eight years old when referred to the Croft to assess whether he had attention deficit syndrome and to look again at his earlier diagnosis of autistic spectrum disorder. Although he was a slow learner he was managing reasonably well in mainstream primary school, but his mother and stepfather were reporting that they were having difficulties managing his aggressive behaviour at home. He had been admitted to the Croft as a day patient for a four-week assessment.

When I went to collect Damien from the classroom for his second individual music therapy diagnostic assessment, he was quiet and compliant and seemed content to come with me. This was the general picture that both I, and other staff on the unit had seen of Damien, a quiet boy who spoke when spoken to but did not tend to initiate conversation or become very animated. In the music therapy group where I had seen him during the previous week, he was quite involved in playing the instruments but generally seemed to fade into the background and not stand out in any way.

In this second diagnostic assessment, in his second week at the Croft, he sat quietly while I sung the 'Hello' song to him and then, when asked to choose what to do next, asked me to play and sing the 'Rainbow' song to him. He joined in quietly at first, singing beautifully in tune. Then when I suggested that he could sing out a little he surprised me by shouting out the words very loudly. When I said that he could do something in between the very quiet singing and the shouting he became very quiet again. I wondered whether he found it hard to operate in a 'middle ground'. Either he became very loud and quite wild or he kept very quiet for fear of losing control. On the unit so far he had only shown us his quiet side.

Towards the end of our session, we improvised a story while accompanying ourselves by free play on the instruments. Damien suggested that the story should be about a naughty boy. He then said that 'he [the boy in the story] smashed a plate' while at the same time hitting the cymbal excitedly. I echoed this response and was then told that 'his mum was very cross' and 'he broke another plate!' with more cymbal crashes. Damien was now very involved and laughing excitedly as the boy in the story smashed the television, pulled down a lamp and caused a power cut. The boy's parents kept being very cross and finally locked him in his bedroom and threw the key away. All the suggestions were coming from Damien, I was mainly confirming and echoing back his ideas. The story went on and on with excited shouts of 'he smashed another plate' every time I tried to encourage Damien to bring the storyline to a conclusion. Finally the tale ended with Father Christmas coming to the house and the boy's behaviour calming down. Damien was also quiet again, showing little sign of having just been shouting excitedly.

I remember feeling both pleased that Damien was using the session to express himself and also uncomfortable at his joy and excitement about imaginary violence and chaos. With Damien and his family's permission we had videotaped the session so I was able to show excerpts of the session to the rest of the staff. The team were amazed to see a completely different side of Damien, but wondered whether he might have witnessed violence at home and was re-enacting scenes in our improvised story. Inquiries were made and it transpired that as a small child he had been present during violent exchanges between his mother's previous partner and his teenage son. This then enabled us to discuss these issues with Damien's family and explain some of his difficulties. In our overall assessment we felt that he did not have attention deficit disorder and that he was only borderline for autistic spectrum disorder.

Clearly the music therapy diagnostic assessment had a key role to play for Damien as it was in this session that he first showed us a different side to his personality and gave us clues about the cause of his difficulties.

Nancy, Claude and Phoebe

Nancy was referred to the Croft with her two children – Claude, aged two and Phoebe, aged 11 weeks – as an inpatient for a parenting assessment. She had suffered postnatal depression after the births of both her children and had been hospitalised for three months after the birth of her first-born. The depression she suffered after Phoebe's birth had been less severe and did not require hospital treatment. She was admitted to the unit so that we could support her in her parenting skills and assess whether she was able to manage.

Nancy clearly cared deeply for her two children and looked after their physical needs in a quiet and efficient way. However, she lacked confidence in her ability to play with them, and remained quite flat in her exchanges with them showing very little emotion and smiling feebly rather than reacting strongly. She tended to retreat to her room in the evening after the children had gone to bed and was shy about talking to other families or staff. The team felt that family music therapy sessions might be a way to help Nancy to have fun and play more spontaneously with her children.

Before taking the three of them to the music therapy room, I explained to Nancy that the aim of the sessions was for all of them to have some fun together through playing the instruments and music making. Nancy agreed to 'give it a try' although she said she was not very musical herself.

I started with my usual 'Hello' song. Claude smiled and cuddled up to Nancy and she responded to this warmly, giving him a hug with one arm while holding baby Phoebe in her other arm. Phoebe was clearly very aware of my singing and playing, her eyes as round as saucers.

I then offered Claude a large drum, which he tapped a few times with his hand. However, he was reluctant to play with a beater, even though Nancy played herself to try to encourage him. It was when Claude saw the reed horn that he really came into his own. He blew down it loudly, laughing delightedly when he made a big sound. I gave Nancy a reed horn of her own to play and picked up my clarinet to improvise around the two reed horn pitches. Soon Claude was blowing down his mother's ear and squealing with pleasure when she laughed and backed away. During these interchanges Phoebe was following what was happening and jigging up and down excitedly. I had never seen Nancy so animated and the two children were obviously thoroughly enjoying their mother's involvement in the game.

After the session, Nancy told me that she had not expected to enjoy it and was pleased to feel she could play instruments with the children. We agreed to video the following week's session so that we could have a record of the three of them having fun together. I also wanted to be able to point out to Nancy how good she was with her children, automatically helping and supporting them in their play. I thought that if she could see herself on video interacting so positively with her children, her confidence in her own abilities would increase. I also thought that, with Nancy's consent, it would be useful to show these sessions to the Croft team as Nancy had not been so animated or engaged in other settings on the unit.

Defining my approach

The foregoing two vignettes show that short-term music therapy interventions have an important and unique role to play within a child and family psychiatric team. Clients show different sides of themselves in musical interactions with the therapist, often becoming more intensely involved and engaged than in other settings. In Nancy's case it was particularly important to help her to focus on, and become aware of, the positive aspects of her interactions with her children.

Although there are many aspects of music making that are therapeutic it is the musical interaction that is at the centre of my work, which is why my approach is called 'interactive music therapy'. In my companion book (Oldfield 2006) I describe my approach in detail and explain how my work has points in common with, and differs from, the work of a number of music therapists. Here I will mention a few points and focus on those aspects that are relevant to my work in child and family psychiatry.

Like Alvin (1966), my method is musical and I use almost exclusively live and mostly improvised music in my sessions. It is through the non-verbal improvised musical exchanges that I can engage and capture children and parents' interest and attention. The music making is a means to an end. The therapeutic objectives are non-musical but the way to engage the client is through the music. However, unlike Alvin, I often work with parents, and I work more closely than she did as a member of the psychiatric team.

Nordoff and Robbins (1977) and Bunt and Pavlicevic (2001) emphasise the importance of the relationship between the client and the therapist, indicating that the focus for therapeutic change lies in this relationship. Most of the work described by these authors is long-term, so the type of relationship I develop in my short-term work in child and family psychiatry will not be the same. In addition, in my work, it is the relationship between the child and the parent that is often the focus of attention.

An aspect of my work that is not so commonly described as essential by other music therapists is the importance of offering children and families a positive experience that they can enjoy. In child and family psychiatry, the music therapy sessions are often the only times that families can tolerate being in one room together, or when children can manage to share in an activity without becoming openly aggressive or distressed.

Within the psychiatric team, my role is often seen as providing a space where children and families can have positive times, be themselves and be listened to both by myself and other members of the family. Other members of the team often expect me to pick up on aspects of children and families that have not been seen elsewhere (as was the case with Damien) and this can then lead to reflection on the possible meanings of these new behaviours or characteristics. Psychodynamic thinking, where we consider the meaning behind behaviours, may help us to understand the children and the families, as well as debates and discussions between different colleagues' interpretations of children's behaviours.

As I explain in my companion book (Oldfield 2006), various psychological theories are relevant to my way of working in child and family psychiatry. Carr's (1999) behavioural approaches are useful particularly when trying to understand children who are struggling to relate to others in positive ways. Some parents, for example, fall into patterns of behaviour where they give their child attention only when the child is in danger or about to cause a problem. Children may then not know how to relate to adults other than through challenging behaviour. These children may reject praise and positive attention from adults partly because this is unfamiliar to them and they do not know how to respond. Similarly children who are on the autistic spectrum may struggle to socialise with their peers. They may have gained attention and respect from other children by being silly and rude to adults, and then develop a pattern of behaving in this way every time they are with their peers, partly because they have not developed any other more positive strategies for socialising.

Winnicott's theories (1960, 1971) regarding the importance of providing emotional support in early childhood, and Stern's ideas on the mother's essential 'affect attunement' (Stern 1985, 1995, 1996), are very helpful when working with children with attachment disorders. Often I find that I am providing non-verbal musical 'nurturing' and 'holding' for both children and parents who have struggled in their early relationships. Some children and parents will be able to use the instruments and improvised exchanges to discover how to play and have dialogue. This was the case for Nancy and Claude who had missed out on these important mother/baby interactions because of Nancy's postnatal depression.

In later chapters I describe my music therapy approach in specific clinical areas and refer to music therapists who have described work in these areas. Overall, if I had to describe my music therapy approach in one sentence I would say that *I have an interactive, positive approach, which involves live and mostly improvised music making.*

Influences from my own background

Coming to work at the Croft Unit after having worked for six and a half years in an institution for 220 adults with learning difficulties was quite a culture shock and somewhat intimidating. The psychiatric unit was much smaller and the staff team were all intense and passionate about their work. They were welcoming and kind but all seemed very knowledgeable. Weekly management meetings were full of lively debates about which approach was appropriate for each child and family. I also came into contact with families who had suffered severe hardships and children who were being abused physically, sexually and emotionally. I became aware of how privileged my own childhood had been and how much I had to learn.

Actually, I think my unusual expatriate childhood in Austria, where I went to a French school but spoke English at home, helped me to cope. Twenty-two years as a foreigner in various countries meant that I knew what it was like to be different and could manage feeling alien somewhat more easily. I was gradually able to take on the unusual role of being a music therapist in this strong team of people. I discovered that I rather enjoyed having a different and specific identity.

Although I had not suffered any hardship as a child, the experience of living in different cultures made it easier for me to identify with families operating in different ways. In spite of my lack of experience regarding deprived and low-income families, I found it quite easy to understand a wide variety of approaches to childcare and family life.

Some thoughts about working in child and family psychiatry

In *Interactive Music Therapy – A Positive Approach* (Oldfield 2006) I explain how I feel about my work as a music therapist with pre-school children with autistic spectrum disorder and their parents. I describe how I consult my previous week's notes and then become completely immersed in that particular child's world. Although every session is different I will work with children and parents for many weeks and our music making will evolve in some predictable ways and special patterns of communication will develop for each family.

At the Croft Unit my work consists partly of two-week diagnostic assessments, an on-going weekly open music therapy group for all the children on the unit, and short-term (usually four to twelve weeks at the most) individual or family music therapy treatment. In the diagnostic assessments, I aim to assess some of a child's strengths and weaknesses in order to assist the team in the diagnostic process. Once my two sessions are completed, I feed back to the team and occasionally suggest a few further individual or family music therapy sessions in order either to focus on assessing a particular area of strength or difficulty or to do some short-term music therapy treatment.

When I arrive for work at the Croft, I often will have no idea at all what to expect and how sessions will go. Most weeks I will see one or two children for the first time. The children I am seeing for the second or third time will often be very different from when I saw them previously, either because the medication they are having has been changed, or because their behaviour may be influenced by new families who have arrived on the unit. When I am working with families, even when I make efforts to plan who will be coming I often do not know ahead of time which family members will be there. One of the most important aspects of the work in this setting is to be flexible and not to get frustrated by unexpected events.

Nevertheless, I find the work at the unit incredibly interesting and exciting. Often the children's behaviours are disruptive and difficult so it is a major achievement sometimes simply to keep all the children in the music group in the room for 40 minutes without any major outbreaks occurring. When in addition to remaining in the room children are clearly enjoying the music making and able to interact in positive ways, I feel a great sense of achievement. Again and again I am struck by how much easier it is for some children to make music together non-verbally than it is to use spoken language.

Every week at the Croft is a challenge. I know that I will not always be able to overcome the difficulties the children and their families present, but I feel it is important to try. In some ways I welcome unpredictable challenges as it is the difficult cases that continue to make the work interesting and exciting even after working at the Croft for 18 years. I think that the fact that I often have to think of new ways of tackling difficult situations enables me to continue to be creative and motivated. If I always knew exactly what to do I might run the risk of becoming stale and boring.

Deep down I know that I can usually do something to help. If I do not manage as well as I would like, I have the back-up and support of an exceptional staff team. Working closely with the Croft team is one of the most rewarding aspects of the work.

Parallels with family life at home

Since I have been working at the Croft Unit, I have had four children. In this and the next section I will explore some of the parallels between my working life and my family life.

My oldest son, Daniel, was born in 1988, 18 months after I started working in child and family psychiatry. I remember being very aware of the fact that I was working with families with relationship difficulties with their children while at the same time looking forward to starting my own family. Clinical supervision sessions helped me to keep my feelings about my own future child separate from my thoughts about the families I was trying to support and help, while at the same time learning from both situations in a positive way.

Going back to work, part-time, four months after Daniel's arrival was a very positive experience. I was delighted to return to work that I loved and to focus on something other than babies and housework. As a mother myself I now felt more confident about supporting mothers who were exhausted after sleepless nights. However, by the early afternoon, I remember looking forward to seeing my baby again and found it was much easier than previously to switch off work and become engulfed by life at home after I collected Daniel from his childminder.

By 1992 I had four children, including twins. Going back to work seven months after the twins were born definitely felt a lot easier than looking after four young children at home. However, after this more prolonged break from work, I wondered whether I would still know how to be a music therapist. Would I still be able to improvise, would I be able to get through to children and families, and was I still capable of doing my job? Discovering that all had not been forgotten was a huge relief. I realised how much I had missed my work and was reminded how inspiring the process of helping people through creative music making was.

Over the years I have found that the combination of raising a family and working as a music therapist has very worked well. Because I am a mother myself I have more confidence to give practical advice or make suggestions to other families. Sometimes, I mention that I have children myself because I feel that it helps families to know that I have first-hand experience of dealing with babies and children. However, I have to be careful not to appear over-confident as that could, for example, be intimidating for a mother with postnatal depression after her first child, faced with a mother of four who appears to be managing well. I try to show that I can empathise with other families' difficulties without indicating that I know all the answers. I also find it is useful to know what can be expected of 'normal' children of different ages and what types of family difficulties are to be expected. Quite frequently in our weekly management meetings at the Croft, staff with primary school children of their own will remind the others that apparently deviant behaviours of children at the Croft are quite 'normal' and to be expected.

The fact that I have learnt to deal with very difficult behaviours from children at the Croft has helped me to be consistent and thoughtful about approaching my own children's difficulties. I have not become a therapist with my own children, but have learnt to think through the way I handle difficult moments. Working with families in crisis at the Croft, I am constantly reminded of how lucky I am. As a result I think I have learnt to truly enjoy the times in my family life when things are going well.

Therapeutic music teaching

Another parallel between life at the Croft and life at home has been the music teaching role that I have had in both places. At the Croft this has occurred when children have expressed a wish to learn to play a tune or a piece (usually on the piano or the xylophone) and I have felt that it would be therapeutic to help them to go through a learning process. At home I have supported my four children through their musical education.

In *Interactive Music Therapy – A Positive Approach* (Oldfield 2006) I explore the similarities between music therapy interactions and interactions between chamber music players. Here I compare music teaching roles at the Croft and with my own children at home.

My therapeutic teaching roles at the Croft have often involved helping a child to learn a tune they have asked me to teach them, such as 'Twinkle,

Twinkle' or the 'Snowman Song' on the piano. Although part of my aim is to help the child to learn how to play and remember the correct notes in the correct rhythm, I will also be concerned with the learning process and how the child is responding to being taught a new skill. Some children will concentrate really hard and persist until the tune has been mastered. Others will focus for a few seconds, do something else and keep coming back to the tune briefly throughout their session with me. Some children will accept guidance from me, others will need to find the correct notes themselves. Some children will use only one finger at first, others will want to label notes with special codes and then write the codes down on a piece of paper. Unlike many piano teachers who develop systems of teaching, my teaching method will be very flexible and be completely modified and adapted to the learning strengths and choices of each individual child. Many of the children will want to perform the pieces they have learnt to parents, staff and peers, and I will try to ensure that this performance becomes a positive confidence-building opportunity.

Other teaching roles I have had at the Croft have included accompanying children on the piano who wish to perform songs or pieces to their peers in the music group. The pieces are usually played on instruments such as the recorder or the xylophone, or occasionally on an instrument the children may have learnt to play prior to admission, such as the flute or the cornet. Occasionally groups of children have opted to put together some group Christmas performances involving improvised stories, percussion instruments and Christmas songs. For me the emphasis is always on how the process of putting together these performances is beneficial to the children, rather than concerns about a polished performance. I remember an eight-year-old girl with Asperger's syndrome quietly singing the 'Snowman Song' accompanied on the metallophone by a six-year-old boy with attention deficit disorder, before a Christmas lunch with children, parents and staff. The mother of the little girl had tears in her eyes as she told me it was the first time her daughter had ever been involved in any Christmas performance. The father of the six-year-old boy was astounded that his son had managed to sit still for 20 minutes.

With regard to my own children, I have encouraged, cajoled and coerced them in daily instrumental practice. I have accompanied them on the piano during practice sessions and in music exams. I have chosen instrument teachers, been part of lessons at first and then played a role in facilitating a positive relationship between the children and individual teachers. I have taken them to music lessons, chamber music groups and music courses, and listened to many concerts and performances. As a parent, I have been concerned about the quality of my children's playing and have wanted to encourage them to strive for excellence. However, even more important has been that they continue to enjoy their music making and remain motivated to continue to progress. I do not want to force feed them into becoming anxious musicians, but hope that by giving them music skills early on they will have opportunities during their lives to enjoy music and music making in a wide variety of ways. Often it has been a juggling act between encouraging them to keep practising and at the same time maintaining their enthusiasm and love of music. I remember playing stamping games up and down the stairs to encourage my four-year-old son to use bigger bow strokes on the violin. With my second son, on one occasion I suggested that he should twirl his double-bass around on the spot at the end of each phrase to try to make him laugh when he was getting frustrated while practising a particularly difficult piece. For my teenage twin daughters the main attraction of Saturday music school at present is the gang of friends that they meet there every week.

There are parallels in my dual roles of therapist and teacher, and of parent and teacher. In the two situations the teaching role is secondary to my principal role of therapist and parent. In both settings my main goal is to maintain the children's enthusiasm for music and to help them to gain confidence and a strong sense of self through their playing. I have found that the flexible teaching approach I have to use with each child at the Croft has helped me to be creative in thinking of different ways of overcoming difficulties encountered by my own children in their practising. Similarly I have learnt hugely from watching my own children being taught music on a wide variety of courses and these ideas have given me new thoughts for my work at the Croft.

The Croft team

As a music therapist in child and family psychiatry I am entirely dependent on the staff team to be able to work effectively. My first point of contact on arrival on the unit is to talk to the nursing team and find out about the children I will be seeing that day. I run the music therapy group with one or two members of staff, jointly planning and reviewing each session before and after the group. During the day I will feed back informally on music therapy sessions, and discussions about children and families always occur.

In the weekly two-hour management meetings all the families will be discussed by the entire team: psychiatrists, a family therapist, specialist nurses, a teacher, classroom assistants, clinical psychologists and music therapists. I find that it is an incredibly interesting and rewarding experience to be part of a diverse group of people who have different spheres of expertise but are all motivated and often passionate about helping the children and families in their care.

Written music therapy reports at the Croft Unit

After every music therapy session at the Croft Unit I write a short paragraph about the session. This is kept in that child or family's nursing folder and contains notes written by the multi-disciplinary team on a daily basis. These notes are available to parents if they wish to read them. Over the years I have found that it is useful to write these notes on a coloured sheet of paper (at present this is pink) so that the music therapy notes can easily be identified within the folder. A blank music therapy note-writing form, as well as examples of these summaries relating to the vignettes earlier in this chapter, appear in Appendices 1, 2 and 3.

When a family is discharged from the unit, each Croft professional writes a report on the work he or she has done and the reports are gathered together to form a discharge package. These documents are sent to the families, the referrer and other relevant organisations such as social services, schools or psychiatric outpatient departments. Examples of reports relating to the two vignettes in this chapter are included in Appendices 4 and 5.

Conclusion

In this chapter I have given an overview of my interactive music therapy approach in child and family psychiatry. I have defined this way of working more generally in a companion book (Oldfield 2006), which focuses on my work at a child development centre. In Chapters 2, 3, 4 and 5 I look at various aspects of my work as a music therapist at the Croft Unit. In Chapters 6 and 7, I examine music therapy research. In Chapters 8 and 9, I reflect on different ways of teaching music therapy skills and on clinical supervision.

Chapter 2

Music Therapy Diagnostic Assessments in Child and Family Psychiatry

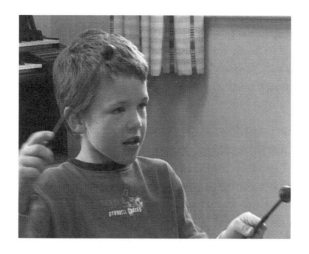

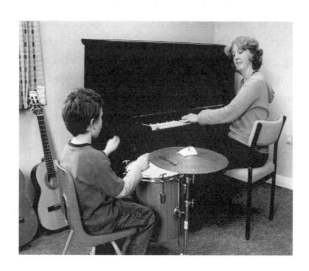

Introduction

In Chapters 2 to 5, I shall be exploring a range of music therapy work in child and family psychiatry at the Croft children's unit. In this chapter, I shall describe the Music Therapy Diagnostic Assessments (MTDAs) that have gradually evolved during my work in this field over the past 18 years. I initially wrote about these MTDAs in Oldfield (2000) and some of the material that follows will be drawn from that article. First, however, alternative approaches will be examined.

Alternative approaches to music therapy assessment

As early as 1971, Nordoff and Robbins wrote:

> The investigational possibilities of music therapy based on improvisation proved to be an aid in differential diagnosis. Comparative experiences made it possible to discern in some children responses that indicated not so much autism as aphasia or brain-injury complicated by emotional disturbance. (p.104)

They then went on to describe a case study where the music therapists' initial diagnostic impressions were shown to have been correct (Nordoff and Robbins 1971, p.104). Not many music therapists have written about this area since 1971, although some have explored music therapy assessments where the aim of the assessment may be to determine whether a client is suitable for music therapy treatment or whether the treatment has been effective.

In 1988, Isenberg-Grezda wrote a review of the music therapy literature on assessment. She concluded that music therapists think of assessment in their work in two ways. The first is part of each music therapist's practice and is an on-going evaluative assessment which consists initially in identifying whether a client will benefit from music therapy treatment, and later in determining the progress made by the client. The second is a diagnostic assessment and consists of comparing the results of music therapy assessments to other assessments and trying to determine what music therapy can offer or add to treatment that is different from other forms of intervention. My work at the Croft clearly comes into the second category described by Isenberg-Grzeda.

In 1993, I wrote an overview of how different music therapists analyse their work and suggested a three-stage assessment procedure which has since been used and adapted by other music therapists (Oldfield 1993a).

This study shows that, although there is no standardised assessment procedure for music therapists, there is an interest in the profession in developing more efficient ways of gathering information about music therapy sessions. This interest in thinking about what information music therapists gather about their clients is perhaps a first step in thinking about whether music therapists could gather information about their clients in different and sometimes more effective ways, other than diagnostic procedures.

It is interesting to note that Nordoff and Robbins developed their music therapy evaluation sheets from scales that were already being used by other staff to evaluate autistic children in a day care centre (Nordoff and Robbins 1977). Scale 1, which was called 'Nature and degree of the relationship to an adult as a person', became the Nordoff and Robbins Scale 1: 'Child–Therapist Relationship in Musical Activity'; and scale 2, originally entitled 'Communication', became the Nordoff and Robbins Scale 2: 'Musical Communicativeness'. Unlike my Music Therapy Diagnostic Procedure and the Autistic Diagnostic Observation Schedule (ADOS) which will be elaborated on in greater depth at a later stage in this book, the scales used in the day centre where Nordoff and Robbins worked were used to evaluate progress made by the children at the centre rather than to diagnose autism. Nevertheless, in both cases the music therapy assessments concentrate on levels of engagement or resistance, and on levels of communicativeness through musical involvement. It is also fascinating to observe that, in both situations, the music therapists successfully adapted an assessment tool that was already in use in the clinical setting.

Wells (1988) described her individual music therapy assessment procedure for young adolescents attending an inpatient psychiatric centre. Three musical tasks were described and their rationales clarified. Each task focused on different areas of assessment, such as level of anxiety, ability to make choices, self-image, attention span and ego boundaries. Assets (or areas of strength) and then 'common musical/behavioural criteria indicators' were described. The primary purpose of this assessment procedure was to ascertain whether music therapy would be a suitable intervention for a client. Although the data collected was reviewed and interpreted, the emphasis was on assessment for music therapy treatment rather than on diagnostic indicators. Nevertheless, it is interesting to note that Wells lists the rationale for musical tasks in a similar way to my description of the 'purpose' of each activity in my sessions at the Croft.

Grant (1995) and Boxhill (1985), two music therapists from the USA, described detailed music therapy assessment procedures. They both argued that music therapists are in a strong position to evaluate the developmentally disabled clients' sensorimotor, perceptual, social and communication skills. The assessments asked large numbers of very specific questions – such as 'Does the client play the resonator bell using mallet while moving horizontally across midline?' – and took several sessions to be completed. These assessments measured the general abilities of clients, and could show progress or deterioration in very specific areas.

In the UK, general levels of ability are usually routinely assessed by psychologists, occupational therapists and physiotherapists, who would each look at even more detailed areas in their own areas of expertise than are covered by Grant and Boxhill. The assessment procedures they described would be too detailed and lengthy for music therapists to use to assess their own work, and only very small parts of the assessments would usually be relevant to individual music therapy clients. In addition, if music therapists attempted to fill in such lengthy and detailed questionnaires about all aspects of the client's development, they would have to completely change the nature of the music therapy sessions and set up test situations where the questions on the assessment forms could be answered. Filling in these types of detailed questionnaire would also detract from the process of 'developing a relationship with the client through spontaneous music making' which tends to be one of the primary concerns of most music therapists working in the UK.

Although in my diagnostic music therapy sessions the aims of my work have to be different from when I am engaged in on-going music therapy treatment, the general approach I have is similar. For example, improvised, spontaneous music making remains at the centre of each session both in music therapy treatment sessions and in diagnostic assessments. In spite of all the differences between the Boxhill and Grant assessment forms and my diagnostic procedures, the core concept that music therapy approaches may be useful to evaluate clients' strengths and difficulties remains similar in both situations.

Loewy (1999) and Rogers (1992) wrote about clinical music therapy situations where new information was revealed to the music therapist. Rogers described long-term individual work with children who had been sexually abused and who sometimes disclosed information in music therapy sessions that had not been shared with other professionals. Loewy worked in a medical centre with chronically ill children and explained how new information about family themes would often be revealed through music therapy sessions. The main way in which this differs from the assessments I am carrying out at the Croft is that new information is gathered incidentally as the therapeutic process evolves rather than being the primary focus of the work. However, their work is very encouraging as it indicates that music therapy can reveal information not revealed in other disciplines or therapies.

Another assessment approach that some music therapists have taken is to analyse the music that comes out of music therapy sessions and compare it with other aspects of the client's strengths and difficulties. Dunachie (1995), for example, was interested in determining whether musical developmental levels matched up with cognitive developmental levels when working with learning disabled adults. Saperston (1999) investigated how developmental singing abilities, object permanence and language development related to one another in young children and adults with learning difficulties. York (1999) developed a 'residual music skills test' to identify the musical skills of people with Altzheimer's disease. Both Saperston and York subsequently used the assessments they had developed as a way of diagnosing the clients' general levels of ability. Here, therefore, we are closer to diagnostic music therapy assessments. The main difference between these approaches and mine is that Dunachie, Saperston and York were measuring musical ability rather than looking at the communication processes that came out of musical improvisations. Because they were focusing on musical ability they had to develop specific musical tests. In a similar way to the assessments by Boxhill and Grant mentioned earlier, the administration of these tests was very different from music therapy sessions, whereas my diagnostic assessments remain very similar to music therapy sessions.

Aldridge (1996) developed 'musical elements of assessment' to help assess receptive and productive areas of functioning for patients with Alzheimer's disease. He also compared features of medical and musical assessments, adapting features of the medical tests to the music therapy situation. For example, 'motivation to complete tasks' could easily be assessed in the music therapy setting by looking at 'motivation to sustain playing'. Although Aldridge was working with a very different client group, the idea of answering questions about levels of ability in the music therapy sessions is not dissimilar to the music therapy assessment investigation I have undertaken in this project.

Wigram (1995) outlined his music therapist assessment work at Harper House where children are diagnosed with a wide variety of conditions such as Rett syndrome, autism and language disorders. His work was similar to my work at the Croft because he was also using music therapy sessions to assist the team in their diagnosis of children who were autistic. He explained that he looked at the way the child responded by asking specific questions under five different headings: general interaction and response, abnormal communication behaviour, musical behaviour, transference of behaviours, or features of pathology into musical behaviour interaction and physical activity and behaviour. Later he gave us a list of approaches and ideas that he used in the sessions. However, at this stage, he did not refer to a specific scoring system or assessment form similar to the systems I have been using at the Croft. This may well be because, as his case studies showed, the range of children seen at Harper House was far more diverse than the children seen at the Croft. It must also be remembered that Harper House is an outpatient clinic whereas the Croft is an inpatient unit. This means that the range of assessments carried out at the Croft will include evening and night-time observations and will generally be more intense than those that can be carried out at Harper House.

A few years later, Wigram (1999, 2000) gave us the model of a structure to his assessment sessions. This model has some similarities to the one I describe both here and in an article (Oldfield 2000). For example, we both include a variety of different musical activities in our sessions which each help us to answer specific questions about the child's strengths and difficulties. In both Wigram's and my work, free and structured musical improvisations play an important part in the sessions. However, Wigram's Improvisation Assessment Profiles (IAPs), which he adapted from Bruscia's IAPs (Bruscia 1987), took the diagnostic process in a very different direction from mine. He explained that he watched the videotapes of each of his assessment sessions and chose selected musical excerpts to analyse in some depth. Wigram's task was not easy, as Bruscia's assessment scales were not intended to be diagnostic procedures but rather assessments of suitability for music therapy treatment or evaluations of progress achieved. However, Wigram's musical analysis of a child's improvised playing reinforced his opinion that the child had a language disorder rather than being on the autistic spectrum. In my work I have avoided purely musical analyses as I have been interested in comparing my assessment procedure with other non-musical assessment systems. I wanted to ask questions that were relevant to the music therapy assessment but could be compared to the questions that were being asked in other diagnostic tests.

In Wigram's most recent article on music therapy assessment (Wigram 2002), he showed a table of an individual child's responses and reactions in music therapy and how these responses related to what he called 'the expectations of therapy' (p.16). The type of information Wigram was collating is similar to the information I am trying to obtain from my MTDAs. However, in my study I have tried to design a test which can easily be compared to the ADOS, and which can be used with all the children who are diagnosed at the Croft, rather than being specific to one child.

Molyneux (2001) used similar music therapy diagnostic assessments to the ones I use at the Croft and described three different assessments where she was able to contribute to the team's evaluations of the children's diagnoses. Molyneux's work is very similar to mine, and she described very positive results, indicating that it was well worth researching this relatively new area of music therapy diagnostic assessments in more depth. This is not altogether surprising as Molyneux trained on the music therapy training course at Anglia Ruskin University and did one of her clinical placements at the Croft.

Although only a few have written about using music therapy directly for diagnostic purposes, many have touched on the subject when describing a variety of different assessment procedures, or when exploring short-term music therapy work. Much of the work described here has had positive outcomes and there seems to be a growing interest in music therapy assessments, short-term music therapy and music therapy diagnostic assessments.

Description of the Music Therapy Diagnostic Assessment (MTDA)

General points

The range of children assessed at the Croft is very wide. Children are referred there for very different reasons. The Croft may, for example, be asked to confirm a suspected diagnosis of attention deficit hyperactive disorder (ADHD), question a diagnosis of autistic spectrum disorder or assess a relationship between a parent and a child. The children's ages range from 4 to 12 years.

The approach to the music therapy assessment obviously varies tremendously depending on each child and family. However, some patterns have emerged over the past few years, which will now be described.

The assessment consist of two half-hour sessions which usually occur at the same time on two consecutive weeks. The staff at the Croft are well-informed about my work. Key workers suggest which children they feel are priorities for music therapy assessments and provide me with basic information about the children and about why they have been referred to the unit. A time is arranged for two assessment sessions and the child is told about the sessions in a morning meeting when the children's timetable for that day is explained. I introduce myself to the child when I go to collect him or her, and we may chat informally as we walk to the music therapy room.

Later in this book I describe a research investigation where I focus on MTDAs for children when there is a possibility that they may be on the autistic spectrum. However, the MTDAs were originally designed to help in the diagnostic process of a wide variety of difficulties typical not only of autistic spectrum disorder but also of attention deficit disorder or Gilles de la Tourette's syndrome, for example. In the research investigation I explain how I developed a scoring system for the MTDAs. I will explore this method of scoring further in the research chapter, and focus here on describing the MTDAs.

The room and equipment

The room is equipped with a piano, an electric organ, several guitars, and a wide range of percussion instruments. I also have a quarter-size violin and bring along my own clarinet. All the instruments are laid out on shelves or stand near the wall and are accessible to the children.

Two small chairs (child size) stand facing one another a little distance from the instruments. Two bigger chairs are in front of the piano. The floor is carpeted and there are a few pictures on the wall: drawings and collages obviously done by children. There is no other furniture except some more stacked-up children's chairs. The room is friendly and spacious but has few distractions. The open shelves covered with instruments invite the child to take an interest in music making. But there is also a sense of tidiness and organisation conveyed by the carefully set out chairs.

Structure of the session

The following is a description of the format I normally use. However, there will always be exceptions and I try to be flexible to meet the needs of each child so that I can create the optimum situation and setting to evaluate a child's strengths and weaknesses.

I invite the child to sit down on the chair facing me, and sit down opposite the child. I say something like: 'Here's a chair for you and I'll sit here', usually gesturing as I speak.

The session begins with a 'Hello' song that I sing to the child, incorporating the child's name and accompanying myself by playing chords on the guitar. The session ends with a percussion duet on the bongo drums where I will sing 'Good bye' and make a clear ending. At some point, either at the beginning or at the end of the session, or as we are walking to or from the music therapy room, I explain that we are having two individual sessions together and remind the child of the time of the session the following week.

In between the 'Hello' and the 'Goodbye', I explain that we will take turns to choose what to do together. This structure is similar in some ways to the on/off approach that I describe in the section 'balance between following and initiating' when writing about my work at the child development centre (Oldfield 2006). At the Croft, this structure gives the children the freedom to choose and make their own decisions. If the process of choosing is too difficult or painful, the child can relax at the times when I provide him or her with my own choices and perhaps a reassuring structure. From the point of view of assessing the child's strengths and weaknesses, I can find out a great deal from the ways in which the child chooses instruments and activities in music therapy sessions. When it is my turn to choose I can set up situations and make suggestions that I feel will give me the maximum amount of information on the way the child is operating and thinking.

For most children, eight or nine of the following activities are included in the MTDA. Activities marked with a star are almost always included in the sessions; three or four of the other activities are chosen depending on each child's preferences and strengths and weaknesses:

- 'Hello' song *
- act of choosing *
- child on large percussion *
- child on wind instrument
- improvised story
- child on violin
- child and therapist play small percussion on floor together

- child and therapist share an instrument such as the bass xylophone or the autoharp
- kazoo dialogue
- piano dialogue
- child and therapist play an instrument each, sitting on chairs *
- child plays electric organ or another instrument and music therapist listens
- therapist teaches child a tune
- 'Goodbye' on bongos. *

The structure of an assessment session could, therefore, take the following form:

1. 'Hello' song on the guitar.
2. Child's choice: child chooses the cabassa and gives me a maraca.
3. My choice: free improvisation; child on drum and cymbal and I play the piano.
4. Child's choice: child chooses piano, I suggest that I play the piano with the child.
5. My choice: a percussion dialogue; I place two slit drums on the floor and we each play them with two beaters.
6. Child's choice: child chooses large bass xylophone, I listen and then join in.
7. My choice: improvised story; child plays metallophone, drum and wind chimes and I go to the piano and we make up a story together.
8. Child's choice: a kazoo dialogue.
9. 'Goodbye' on the bongo drums.

This is quite a large number of activities for any one session. I find that some children who are very well focused will prefer to spend longer on fewer different activities, which sometimes allows us to explore musical improvisations in greater depth. Other children, however, will quickly lose interest and need to move quickly from one thing to the next.

I will now describe each of these headings and then explain what type of information I can gain from each of the musical interactions.

'Hello' song

The 'Hello' song (see Appendix 6) is a gentle, lilting song in 3/4 time, which I sing to the child accompanying myself with chords on the guitar. I include the child's name in the song and will vary the style, speed and length of the song depending on the age of the child and on the way the child is responding to being sung to. I sit opposite the child singing directly to him or her, but again I may turn my chair slightly or face another direction if I sense that this direct contact is overwhelming or very uncomfortable for the child. If I feel that the child is acutely embarrassed, I may make the song very short and make a comment like: 'It's a little strange being sung to like this, isn't it? We'll now move on.'

This beginning has many functions. It establishes straight away that I am going to be actively involved in playing myself and am not just going to listen to the child performing to me. I can observe the emotional response (or lack of response) that the child may have to direct adult warmth and affection. The child may show embarrassment or pleasure, or may reject me by putting hands to his or her ears or turning away. Some children will find it difficult to listen to even a short song and want to get up and find their own instrument or strum the strings while I am playing. Other children will immediately want to inform me of past musical moments in their life or start fantasising about making up their own band. I can observe whether the child's emotional response seems usual or unusual and whether the child has particular difficulties listening or focusing.

The children's choices

After the 'Hello' song I stand up to put the guitar against the wall and I explain that we will take turns to choose what we do in this session. If I feel that the child needs direction I may then say that I will choose first. Otherwise I will ask the child 'Would you like to choose first?' Some children will be quite happy choosing an instrument for each of us and will be uninhibited about improvising freely with me.

Others will go enthusiastically to the piano, the guitar or the bass xylophone and then look bewildered and say 'But I don't know how to play'. It may then be possible to demonstrate that we can improvise freely together, but some children will remain too worried about playing 'properly' to allow themselves to play freely in any way.

For some children, choosing in a musical context is associated with singing songs or learning to play a piece of music on the recorder, and their first choice will be a particular song they want to sing or a piece they want to play on the recorder. If a child chooses to perform to me, I am quite happy to accompany a child singing a nursery rhyme or listen to a piece performed on the recorder. If this is the way the child chooses to start interacting with me musically, I feel a lot can be learnt from listening. The child is sharing a part of his or her musical past with me and this in itself may be revealing and interesting. Similarly, if a child chooses to learn a new piece on the piano or the xylophone, I can discover how the child learns, how tolerant he or she is of personal mistakes, how realistic he or she is about the learning process, and how easily and quickly he or she assimilates new information.

Some children are unable to make choices at all and will say 'I don't know, you choose.' Depending on how anxious I sense the child is at this point, I may be insistent on the child making a choice. I may help the child by saying 'OK, which of these two instruments do you think I might like best?', or I may take over by saying 'Well, if you were able to choose I think you might want to choose this.' If the child is clearly making a point of being defiant, or deciding not to conform, I might go to the piano and say 'You seem to be cross about being here, so I'll play some music myself and try to play in the way that I think you feel.'

Free improvisation

I place the drum and the cymbal in front of the child and then go to the piano. I usually leave time for the child to begin the playing, but if the child is clearly waiting for me then I will start the playing. Some children will look bewildered and be concerned about 'how' they should play. In this case I might say something like 'You can play any way you like; let's see what happens.' During the improvisation I will observe in detail how we are playing together. Because I am assessing the child's needs I will be challenging at times, stopping suddenly perhaps or deliberately changing the style of music we are playing in order to observe how the child reacts. At some point I will usually include pre-composed songs I think the child may have heard before, such as nursery rhymes or theme tunes from children's television programmes. I also try to take note of how the child's playing is making me feel. Do I feel excluded, excited, bored? Is the improvisation enjoyable?

Free improvisations are very useful to find out how a child communicates non-verbally. Does the child initiate ideas or simply copy my suggestions, or do we exchange ideas equally? Do I get the impression that the child is trying to be in control, or does he or she seem desperate for me to lead the activity? Do obsessive, repetitive patterns develop in the child's playing? Do I get the impression that the piece is stuck and that we cannot move on and be creative? Is the child able to enjoy playing freely, or do I feel that the child is getting through some sort of ordeal? Is the child able to listen as well as play? Does the child appear confident or ill at ease? Does the child seem to be expressing feelings in his or her playing? Is the child able to be creative or imaginative?

Answers to all these questions will give me a good idea of how a child communicates non-verbally. Sometimes the patterns of communication will match up to and confirm what other staff on the unit have noticed about a child's verbal communication. But I often notice aspects of communication that have not been observed by other members of staff in different settings. I also think that music therapy assessments sometimes enable me to find out about intricate patterns of communication more quickly than other staff can in different settings.

Percussion dialogues

Percussion dialogues, which could be on any combination of untuned instruments, allow me to confirm the answers to all the questions I was asking in the previous section. In addition I will be able to assess how easily a child shares an instrument and takes turns. I will also find out how playful a child can be and whether a child initiates games or is intent on 'catching me out'. In this more intimate improvisation I will be able to gauge how wary a child is and whether he or she is able to trust and enjoy being with an adult who is not known well.

As Daniel Stern remarked in a paper he gave at the World Congress of Music Therapy in Hamburg in 1996, these types of exchange are very similar to the types of babbling exchange that take place between a mother and a young baby (Stern 1996). For a variety of reasons many of the children I see at the Croft may have missed out on these types of exchange with their own mother, and through percussion exchanges I can evaluate whether a child is able or willing to communicate in this way.

Improvised story

I place a number of large instruments – such as the drum, the metallophone and the wind chimes – in front of the child and then I go to the piano. We start playing together freely, and then I say, 'Let's make up a story. Once upon a time there was a…'. In many cases the child will complete my sentence and say '…a dog!' We improvise together and I say '…where did the dog go?' and the story evolves accompanied by both our improvisations.

Sometimes I have to encourage a child to get going by saying, 'Was it a dog or a cat?' for example. If the child starts a well-known story such as 'Once upon a time there were three bears', I might attempt to change things a little by saying something like '…and they lived in a castle with a magician.' Although spontaneous story-telling could be assessed without the improvised music making, the playing will often motivate a child and fuel his or her imagination. Acting out the story on the instruments makes the story more exciting, and I can improvise on the piano to underline or contain emotions such as excitement, fear or happiness.

These improvised stories combined with music making allow me to evaluate whether the child can make up a coherent story, whether the child allows me to contribute, and whether the child is imaginative or gets stuck in obsessive repetitions or fixed storylines. The child will often become very involved in a story, and will show emotions that have not come to the fore in other settings on the Croft Unit. Sometimes children indirectly share fears or worries with me in these stories that shed light on previously unknown traumas in their life.

Kazoo dialogue

Children frequently will pick up a kazoo from a shelf and ask me what it is and how to play it. I show them and then often encourage the child to choose a kazoo for each of us to play, sitting on the chairs facing one another.

Children sometimes initially find kazoos difficult to play because they blow down them rather than vocalising into them. I try to demonstrate by making 'too too' train-like sounds, 'tweety bird' sounds or singing tunes. Once the child has got the idea we are usually able to have a kazoo dialogue which is often humorous and ends up with both of us laughing. Many children seem to particularly enjoy the fact that we are using our voices to communicate, but that by using sounds rather than words we are equal partners, rather than an adult with extensive vocabulary and knowledge and a child with fewer skills.

Kazoo dialogues are incredibly useful because I can assess how a child responds to different emotions expressed vocally, but without using words. Some children will respond if my vocal sounds are angry or pathetic, but will not take any notice if my vocal sounds become sad. Some children who have very flat, unemotional speaking voices will surprise me by responding very emotionally in kazoo dialogues. Conversely, children who appear to be expressing themselves in ordinary ways through words may be incapable of responding in an emotional way in non-verbal kazoo communication.

'Goodbye'

The goodbye activity on the bongo drums allows me to round off the session. I can evaluate how the child deals with sharing an instrument with me and how he or she copes with close physical proximity. I will have another chance to observe the mother/baby type of non-verbal exchanges mentioned previously. I will also be able to observe whether the child has difficulties with endings, both musical endings and the end of the session.

Feeding back to the rest of the team

It should be obvious from the above description that there is no shortage of information to be gathered from the two diagnostic music therapy sessions. It is important for me to select those pieces of information that will be of greatest interest to the team when feeding back in management meetings. I listen first to what the key workers, the teacher and the other specialists think about a particular child, and then I select pieces of information from my music therapy sessions that seem to shed a new or different light on a child's strengths or weaknesses. In some cases, but in surprisingly few, my observations will confirm what the rest of the team think, in which case I may give a few examples of events to back up the opinions of my colleagues.

Three vignettes

Wayne

Wayne was ten years old and had a previous diagnosis of ADHD as well as a history of difficulties in social interactions. He attended mainstream school where he was allocated a few hours of Learning Support Assistant (LSA) time to assist him with his mild learning difficulties. He was admitted to the Croft Unit because there were concerns from professionals and his family that some of his behavioural difficulties reflected those on the autistic spectrum.

In his first MTDA session Wayne was quiet, lacked spontaneity and seemed to struggle to have fun. However, he made clear choices of what he wanted to do and told me about past musical experiences when he had played his sister's recorder. He had a strong sense of rhythm and was able to have improvised musical exchanges with me where he made musical suggestions as well as picking up suggestions that were made to him.

Wayne was much more at ease in the second MTDA session. He made many spontaneous suggestions and initiated musical ideas. He gradually picked up the idea of having kazoo dialogues with me, changing his vocal intonation and copying and initiating changes of emotion in the vocalisations. Wayne could make only very simple contributions to the improvised musical story, but he did manage to give the story an ending.

In both the MTDA sessions, it was difficult, at times, to understand what Wayne was saying and I was never quite certain whether he had understood what I was saying.

When reviewing Wayne's case during management meetings, the team generally felt that he was autistic. Nevertheless, the changes I had seen in him from one MTDA session to the next indicated to me that, once he was at ease with the situation, he was able to be communicative in non-verbal ways and could even initiate interactions and be quite spontaneous and creative. I suggested to the staff team that his language difficulties might be partly responsible for his social difficulties. In the end we gave him a borderline autistic spectrum diagnosis, rather than an autism diagnosis.

Stuart

Stuart was 12 years old with a history of long-term difficulties in both learning and school. He had been excluded from school many times and over the past year it had become extremely difficult to contain his aggressive outbursts at home. He was admitted to the Croft Unit for an overall psychiatric assessment.

Stuart was initially reluctant to come to music therapy sessions possibly because he had had a previous negative experience related to music. After much negotiation and several missed sessions he finally agreed to come for 15 minutes but did not want to be videoed.

During his first session he was very anxious. He accepted my first suggestion and played the drum and the cymbal very loudly while I accompanied him on the piano. He seemed to enjoy the volume of noise he was generating and briefly allowed himself to enjoy the fact that I was playing loudly *with* him. In general, however, I felt that he was playing for himself while watching how I would react to his loudness rather than using the playing to communicate with me in any way.

After this, Stuart chose a series of percussion instruments in a somewhat frantic and repetitive way, taking very little notice of my musical responses to his playing. He seemed anxious and concerned about being in control of the session. He became quite agitated and refused to accept my suggestions or conform to the structure of the session which involved taking turns to choose what instruments we should play. After ten minutes in the music room he walked out without warning, went to the toilet and then went back to the schoolroom. Later, I talked to him, telling him that I did not mind him leaving the session but that it would be helpful to let me know when he wanted to leave so we could end the session together.

A week later, Stuart was much calmer about coming to the session and consented to come without any fuss. He asked me not to sing the 'Hello' song so I said 'hello' instead and explained that we would again take turns to choose what instruments we would play. This time, Stuart stayed for 15 minutes and asked to finish the session, accepting to play the bongos briefly with me to round off the session. Stuart was calmer during the session, and seemed less desperate about being in control. Nevertheless, I still felt that we were playing in parallel rather than using the music making to give and take or communicate in any way.

Stuart was very difficult to manage on the unit and had to have an individual programme because he refused to take part in any activities with the younger children on the unit. In general, the staff team felt that Stuart had a conduct disorder. However, when I suggested that he might have some deep-seated difficulties in communicating that might often be masked by his general anxiety and disruptive behaviours, he was given an ADOS test which revealed that he was borderline autistic spectrum disorder in addition to having a conduct disorder.

Deborah

Deborah was a four-year-old and had been known to the psychiatric service for a year before her admission to the Croft Unit. There had been concerns regarding unpredictable, confrontational behaviour both at home and at nursery. She was admitted to the Croft with her mother with a query regarding autistic spectrum disorder or ADHD. As Deborah was only four years old it was agreed that I should see her with her mother.

Deborah was pleased to come into the room and wanted her mother to join in with the playing. She had very clear ideas about what she wanted to play but was also able to accept suggestions from myself as well as from her mother and to conform to the clear structure of the music therapy session. There were times when it felt as though Deborah wanted to be in control and was trying to draw her mother into conflict. Nevertheless, Deborah responded well to praise and could be distracted from getting stuck in an argument.

Deborah showed a lovely sense of imagination, pretending to drive a bus while playing the ocean drum and encouraging mother and me to sing songs on the bus. At other moments she seemed quite immature, saying 'me do it' in a toddler-like way.

Deborah was very motivated to play most of the instruments but had obvious difficulties holding on to two beaters and co-ordinating her movements. At times she was also quite distractible, often fiddling with a second instrument while still playing the first one. In our musical improvisations, Deborah was communicative and playful and it was possible to take turns and exchange ideas.

In her two MTDA sessions with her mother, I felt that Deborah presented me with a very mixed picture. On the one hand she was social and communicative, showing imaginative and creative play; on the other hand, she seemed to feel a need to be in control and found it hard to relax into communicative exchanges. At times, I felt that she was very engaged with me and was communicating intensely with both her mother and me. At other times she found it hard to focus and maintain her interest in what we were doing.

On the unit Deborah clearly struggled in group situations, showing few spontaneous overtures to other children and sometimes needing very clear boundaries not to be aggressive to other children. She was given a diagnosis of Pervasive Developmental Disorder of a non-specific type (PDD-NOS) which I felt reflected some of what I had seen in my MTDA sessions. However, I did not really feel that the intense communicative exchanges I had had with her were typical of autistic spectrum disorder. Two years later I found out that she had been seen again in the outpatient service. She had started to have vocal tics and her diagnosis was changed from PDD-NOS to Tourette's syndrome.

Conclusion

In this chapter I have described the MTDAs that have been developed at the Croft Unit. I have also argued that MTDAs are a relatively new development in the profession. In the next chapter I shall focus on a music therapy group I have run at the Croft for many years and which also helps in the assessment and diagnosis of the children's difficulties.

Chapter 3

Music Therapy at the Croft: Assisting Clinical Diagnosis

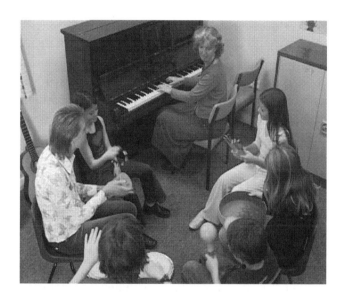

Introduction

I have run a music therapy treatment group at the Croft Unit for Child and Family Psychiatry since September 1987. From 1995 the Croft began to focus on assessment work rather than long-term treatment. The music therapy group has reflected these changes by developing an approach aimed at using the group to assist the team in their diagnostic process. In 2002 my colleague Emma Davies (née Carter) and I wrote an article about this for a book on music therapy groups (Carter and Oldfield 2002). Some of the material from that chapter is used here, along with additional activities and case studies. The first three case studies were written by Emma Davies when she ran the group at the Croft for three years while I was doing my PhD research. These case studies were originally written to be part of the joint chapter we wrote in 2002 but were not included in the final version.

Although a number of music therapists such as Hibben (1991), Tyler (2001) and Molyneux (2001) have written about music therapy groups with children, none of this literature describes work that is specifically to aid diagnosis. This is partly why I have devoted a whole chapter to the topic.

General organisation of the music therapy group

The session takes place every week at the same time and lasts one hour. It is an open group in that all the children who are on the unit are expected to take part. However, occasionally children may be unable to tolerate being in groups at all or may find a whole hour in a group too long. If a child is experiencing particular difficulties remaining in the group, this is discussed with the child prior to the session and a strategy is worked out. This may involve letting an adult know that they need to leave the room, or positioning them near the door and agreeing that if they are finding it difficult to manage, they may leave quietly, with the knowledge that a member of staff will be outside to support them.

I run the group with a member of the Croft nursing team who chooses to work with this group on a regular basis and his or her shifts are worked out accordingly. In addition, there is a named back-up person in case the regular co-worker is unavailable or in case it is felt that an additional member of staff is necessary. The co-worker and I meet before every session to plan, and after every session to review the work. Although I will be running the session and my co-worker will often be supporting the children in their playing while I might be playing the piano, for example, I consider that our roles are of equal importance and we both need each other to run the session. If I am absent the co-worker and the back-up member of staff run a group in the music therapy room with the children, sometimes using excerpts of recorded music. They explain to the children that the group will be different, but this arrangement means that some continuity is maintained even when I am absent.

The session is held in the music room at the Croft. This room is well equipped with a piano, an electric organ and a wide variety of simple percussion and wind instruments as well as some instruments from different countries. The children are brought to the room by the co-worker and another member of the nursing team. I set up the right number of chairs in the room and welcome the children into the room. At the end of the session, the music therapist and the co-worker take the children back to the living area of the Croft where the children get ready to have their lunch.

Most of the children who attend the group will also have individual music therapy assessments with me. This does sometimes affect the work that goes on in the group, and any issues can be addressed either in the individual or in the group sessions.

Group philosophy

Some of these points will be similar to ideas presented in my previous book (Oldfield 2006), while others will be more specifically relevant to working with the particular client group in child and family psychiatry.

The group music therapy session at the Croft aims to provide another forum in which the children's strengths and difficulties can be assessed. The children vary in age from 5 to 12 years and have a wide variety of skills. Some children will be new to the group and the Croft, others will know the unit and will have very clear expectations. At all times, I have to keep the individual needs of each child in mind as well as being conscious of the needs of the group as a whole. This can be a great challenge and it is essential that I liaise closely with both the group co-worker and other members of the Croft team in order to be aware of new abilities or difficulties that have emerged since the previous week's session. It is also important for me to be aware of the group climate at the Croft. There might be, for example, particular rivalries that have developed amongst the children or a generally low or very excited feeling in the group.

Many of the children on the unit lack confidence and have very low self-esteem. I always make a point of emphasising positive aspects of the children's behaviour in the group and try to avoid focusing on difficult behaviours. If children behave in ways that are dangerous to themselves, to other people, or to the equipment in the room, then it is sometimes necessary to exclude them. Nevertheless, an effort is always made to re-integrate the children into the group in as positive a way as possible.

Occasionally my co-worker and I might disagree on the correct way of dealing with one child's behaviours. The way a disciplinary problem is dealt with in the music therapy group may be different from the way the same problem is dealt with in other situations on the unit. When this occurs, it is essential that the issue be discussed between us and a compromise may have to be agreed on, in the best interest of each particular child. For example, some children will be able to manage different rules in different groups whereas others will find this too confusing. The important issue is that the children are aware that staff talk to one another and are all attempting to understand and help as much as they can.

The dynamic structure of our group is as follows. I am clearly in charge, suggesting activities and outlining group rules for different types of music making. However, I will also listen carefully to musical and verbal suggestions made by the children and constantly pick up ideas and suggestions from the children. It is essential that the children in the group feel listened to. When possible I involve the children in choices and decisions regarding the musical activities. At times, my co-worker and I make a point of discussing a contentious group issue openly within the group setting, showing that these issues are considered carefully and not the sole responsibility of one adult. When boundaries have to be set, my co-worker and I try to explain why these limitations are being imposed. At times it might be useful to involve the children in discussion about why adults set boundaries.

My co-worker and I often demonstrate and model activities rather than giving lengthy verbal explanations. The children will usually be drawn into music making in a playful way rather than through a reflective analytic process. Nevertheless, the sessions will always be reviewed very thoroughly and it is at this point that the children's interactions may be examined in a more thoughtful and sometimes analytical way.

Rationale for the group

The reasons for including this music therapy assessment group in the children's weekly programme are similar to the rationale for music therapy in general, outlined in Chapter 1. Here I will outline some aspects that seem particularly important for a group in children with psychiatric needs.

Motivation

In general, many children with psychiatric needs lack confidence, are low in mood and can be difficult to engage in activities. However, the children are usually very motivated to play the instruments and be part of the music making process. The music group is usually a group that the children want to be in, and it is partly because of the children's high level of motivation that this group provides the staff joining in the session with an excellent additional opportunity to evaluate the children's strengths and difficulties. Many children will be excited by playing as a group and easily drawn into group crescendi and accelerandi. Sometimes children will lack confidence to play on their own but will be happy to play as part of a group, where the particular sound they are making blends into the whole and does not stand out.

Music making can provide a non-verbal way of communicating through sound
Some children with language difficulties will enjoy and feel at ease with the fact that music making allows them to make sounds and express themselves without the need to use language. Spontaneous musical turn-taking and exchanging can be satisfying and yet simple to understand and follow. When leading a group improvisation I can include all the children in the group equally, even if some are playing at a more sophisticated level than others.

Music making can provide an opportunity to explore issues of control
Many children at the Croft have behaviour difficulties and a large portion of these difficulties centre around the balance of control between a child and his or her parents or between a child and teachers.

Although I will very clearly lead and organise the group, the musical control can very subtly be shifted from the music therapist to individual children or to the group as a whole. This allows me to give individual children varying amounts of control, which may be very challenging for some children and very rewarding for others. Children can be observed in leading and following roles, and I can push or reassure children depending on individual strengths.

The music therapy assessment group is structured, predictable and safe
The fact that music happens in time and that songs have a clear beginning and end means that music making can be reassuring for children who are constantly seeking for reassuring structures in their life. Of course, much of the music played in these groups is unpredictable and improvised. Nevertheless it is not without form and I usually make sure pieces have clear, well-defined endings. It is also possible to experiment with musical structures and see how free the children can be in their playing. However, it is always possible for me to return to a leitmotiv or a familiar tune if I feel that a particular child needs to be reassured.

Group structure

I will now describe a selection of group activities and then explain how each activity helps us to assess the children's strengths and difficulties. I will describe more activities than I would ever include in one group to illustrate the wide range of things that I might do. Some of these activities will be suitable for older or younger children, and I might also use activities that I have described for music therapy groups at a child development centre (Oldfield 2006).

The number of activities included in each group varies tremendously. Sometimes children take a long time over two or three activities and time is spent talking and reflecting on what we have been doing. At other times, the children need to move quickly from one thing to another and a choice is then made often spontaneously as to the most appropriate activities to suggest. This depends very much on the children and the difficulties they are experiencing. Thought is also given to making them gender-, culture- and age-appropriate. Some of these activities are chosen or adapted from the book *Pied Piper* (Bean and Oldfield 2001). Sometimes children will have their own suggestions and ideas for an activity. Care is taken to incorporate these into the group whenever possible.

In addition to the diagnostic considerations, I must be aware of balancing the needs of individual children with the needs of the group as a whole. Thus an activity may be chosen to reassure a child with obvious low self-esteem, for example, rather than purely for diagnostic purposes. Another consideration will be the contrast and balance of one activity with another. For instance, an activity that involves free movement around the room may be suggested after an activity involving intense concentration. This can provide the children with an opportunity to let off steam. The purpose here is to structure activities to maintain the children's interest. Obviously the diagnostic process will be enhanced if the children remain engaged, so it is important to keep this factor in mind as well as considering which types of activity will allow the most effective observation of the children's strengths and weaknesses.

It is also important to remember that although the structure of the session and the activities suggested are central to the organisation of the group, these activities are only vehicles through which the adults assess the children's strengths and difficulties. My approach to the running of the group is flexible, according to the particular needs of the children, and may involve introducing ideas that have come to me on the spur of the moment.

Verbal introduction

DESCRIPTION

I explain that this is the music group and that it lasts one hour and happens at the same time each week. It is also explained that there are two rules in the music room: first the instruments are not to be damaged; and second, people must not hurt each other or themselves. Sometimes these rules will be mentioned at the start of the session, but at other times they will be implied rather than stated. For some children with conduct disorders, laying down rules at the beginning of a session could be seen as a challenge to attempt to contravene these rules and might actually encourage children to exhibit challenging behaviours. For other children it will be important to have these rules clearly stated so that a safe and reassuring environment is created.

Sometimes, I also explain that all the children will have the opportunity to have a free choice at the end of the session, which means that they will be able to choose any instrument and play it to the rest of the group. This is often something that the children look forward to and can act as a motivator to manage difficult moments during the session. Nevertheless there are some children who would not be able to listen to other children for more than a minute or two without doing something themselves, so there may be times when definite free choices may not be an option in the session.

PURPOSE

The verbal introduction helps to give the group an identity of its own and inform the children that they will have a chance to choose an instrument at some point in the session. Old group members can be given responsibility, which may help them to welcome new children to the group. The old children's enthusiasm for the group will also reassure new children about the value of the group. By encouraging the children to help each other, I give them some responsibility for the running of the session. This gives the children a chance to feel that it is their group, rather than just another occasion where they are expected to do as the adults say.

Introduction / 'Hello' song

DESCRIPTION

The group always begins with a 'Hello' song (see Appendix 6). Sometimes old group members will be invited to tell newcomers how this initial activity works. I sing the 'Hello' song, accompanying myself with the tambourine, and then pass the tambourine to one of the children in the group. During the singing the rest of the group are encouraged to copy the rhythm of the song, which will vary and change in order to ensure that the children are watching and listening. The child who receives the tambourine then plays it and sings or says the song. Then this child will be copied by the rest of the group and may enjoy trying to catch out other group members by playing in unexpected ways. The tambourine is then passed on to the next child.

PURPOSE

This is a clear way to start. It helps the children to settle and to understand that this is now the beginning of the music group. It is also a way of learning each other's names, of introducing each other musically, rather than verbally, which some children find easier. However, some children will struggle to make eye-contact with their peers and show little facial expression.

From this simple activity it is possible to observe whether a child can make choices, whether the music engages the child and holds his/her attention, and whether the child is able to wait, listen and take turns. Sometimes children are reluctant to say their own names and will just beat, or even just hold the tambourine. Other children will refuse to have a turn at all. This could show that a child lacks confidence or has little sense of self. Some children will be reluctant to follow their peers' beat and feel a need to be constantly in control. Emotionally needy children might always choose adults to pass the tambourine on to and may generally be very attention seeking.

Passing the tambourine around in a variety of ways
DESCRIPTION

After the 'Hello' song I might suggest that the tambourine be passed around in a variety of different ways, such as pretending it is very hot, sticky, heavy or asleep (which would mean that it had to be passed around quietly so that it does not wake up). Sometimes I ask the children for their ideas.

PURPOSE

This activity easily involves the children and makes them feel that they have some input into the group, yet at the same time they know that the adults are in control, which is an important feeling for many of the children at the Croft. From this activity the adults in the group can observe whether a child is able to use his or her imagination and play this game, and also see whether the child expresses any positive responses if praised for being especially imaginative.

Passing a sound around

DESCRIPTION

A large instrument such as a drum or a cymbal on a stand is placed in the middle of the circle. The group sits around the instrument just near enough to be able to reach the edge with their fingers. Someone plays the instrument with the tip of a finger in front of a child. That child then plays in front of another child, and so on. I usually model this activity by first passing the sound to my co-worker who might pass the sound back to me before I then pass the sound to a child whom I feel will quickly understand what we are doing. The challenge is for the sound to pass around quickly, without any talking.

PURPOSE

This idea involves an element of choice and surprise and the children usually enjoy the challenge of passing around the sound as fast as possible. Children will sometimes pair up and keep passing the sound to one another. Occasionally the group will attempt to exclude a particular child, or the children will gang up to exclude the adults. These tactics can be commented on by the adults, or ignored depending on the particular difficulties of each of the children. We can observe how children react to these types of exclusion, and issues of bullying or being bullied might be aired. I will make sure that nobody is really upset if they are being excluded and often comment positively when children are clearly helping and supporting one another.

Choosing musical instruments

DESCRIPTION

There are a variety of ways in which the instruments can be chosen. I often suggest that the children close their eyes and one child chooses instruments for each of the children in the group and places them under the children's chairs. The job of distributing the instruments can be offered as an incentive to a child who is finding the beginning of the group difficult to manage, or to make a child's final group special.

PURPOSE

This activity allows the adults to observe whether children are able to close their eyes, wait and remain in their seat. It is also possible to see whether there is any excitement at the prospect of having something chosen for them, and also whether they are able to tolerate an instrument being chosen that is not of their liking. For the child who is choosing instruments, we can see whether he or she is able to risk making decisions and taking responsibility. It is also interesting to observe what instruments children choose, both for each group member and for themselves, as it can be an indicator of how they perceive themselves and others within the group or how they would like to be perceived. For example, in a recent group, a child chose very small instruments (Indian bells, castanets and a thumb piano) for the other children, but chose bongo drums for herself. It may be interesting to note that she was the only girl in a group of four boys.

Group playing
DESCRIPTION

When I start playing the piano, the children are encouraged to pick up their instruments and play freely. When the piano playing stops, they are asked to place their instruments carefully under their chairs before moving round to the chair on their left. I often emphasise how quietly some children have managed to put their instrument under their chair, asking them to do it again while the whole group listens carefully. All the time I am aware of the children's different abilities and needs. For example, I might challenge a very able child to put the ocean drum under her chair which both the child and I know is almost impossible. On the other hand I might make a big fuss about how quietly a less able six-year-old had managed to put a tambour under his chair. Most weeks I will insert well-known tunes into my piano-playing and encourage children to identify which tunes have been played before moving around to the next seat. Again I work around the different ages and abilities in the group by encouraging children who always immediately guess tunes to give the others clues, or mouth the song without any noise, for example.

At times, various aspects of this activity have become increasingly competitive with children insisting they have 'won' and others finding this difficult to accept. Children may have to be encouraged to accept the fact that they cannot always win but that they may have a chance next time. Where possible I try to help the more able children to feel good about themselves by giving them praise and responsibility, so that they do not feel a need to emphasise that they are better, or quicker, than the others.

PURPOSE

Some children are very competitive and become upset when they feel they are not winning or achieving better than their peers. This is particularly the case for some children when they first start in the group. As they begin to feel more at ease in the sessions they can sometimes relax and enjoy the playing without feeling desperate about competing with their peers. The group playing enables us to observe how children interact with their peers and how confident they feel in relation to the other children.

Inserting familiar tunes allows me to introduce reassuring structures at the same time as picking up and following different children's style of playing. It will be possible to observe whether a child is embarrassed by hearing nursery rhymes that are usually associated with younger children or whether he or she does not appear concerned by this issue. Some children obviously love having a chance to be 'little' whereas others dismiss such songs as babyish.

The group playing provides a forum for assessing how engaged and motivated the children are in playing their instrument with others, whether they play in an isolated way or whether they appear aware of what the rest of the group (including the therapist at the piano) is doing. It is also possible to observe whether children can listen to and carry out instructions, and therefore what their level of comprehension is.

Coded instruments

DESCRIPTION

Before the children come into the room a small piece of paper folded in four is placed on their chairs. I explain that the pieces of paper each have a secret code on them that the children must remember without telling the others. The codes will be a variety of shapes such as a circle, a triangle, a cube, a star etc. After the preliminary introductory activities, and perhaps a little bit of group playing, I turn to the group and show them a piece of paper with three or four shapes on it. I tell the children that only those whose secret codes are on the piece of paper should play. Quite quickly I show the children a series of pieces of paper with different combinations of shapes on them. I then ask everyone to put their instruments down and ask the children to tell me what codes their peers have each been given. Some children are usually much better at this than others but I can usually integrate everyone in this game in some way.

PURPOSE

This is a good activity for capturing the attention of those children who are easily bored and struggle to focus. Sometimes children who were not thought to be very able surprise us by being very good at working this game out. Again we can assess whether children have the confidence to keep trying or lose heart when they start feeling they are no good at something. Some children will find it impossible to keep their code secret and will make other children cross by trying to peep at pieces of paper. Other children will team up and beat the system by helping each other. Much can be found out about how the children operate as a team in this game, even if the code breaking does not always go according to the original plan.

Breaking the code
DESCRIPTION

My co-worker and I agree on a code regarding how we are going to respond to one another musically. For example, I play a few beats on my end of bongo drums we hold between us. If I look straight at my co-worker she copies what I have done. If I look away, she plays something different. We play a duet to the group responding to one another in this way and then ask the group to guess what our code is. We then get the children to team up in pairs, make up their own code and play it to the group for the others to guess. As they prepare their duets the adults go around the group supporting the children and making helpful suggestions where necessary.

PURPOSE

This can be a challenging activity for slightly older children. We can assess how children work together and whether they can plan constructively. Some children will be less shy playing to the group as part of a decoding game than if they were asked to play an instrument for everyone to listen to. We can also assess how creative and adventurous children are and whether they are confident enough to take risks.

Eye conducting
DESCRIPTION

I place three small instruments on the floor in the centre of the circle, about a metre away from each other. I then ask the children to look at my eyes and emphasise that this is an activity where we do not talk at all. I look very clearly at my co-worker (or a child who is familiar with this game) and then look down at one of the three instruments, indicating with my head that the instrument should be picked up. As soon my co-worker has picked up the instrument I jig and wriggle on my chair indicating that the instrument should be played. I will stop and start moving clearly to indicate stops, and the speed of my movements will indicate how energetically and fast the instrument should be played. I will then indicate that the instrument should be put down and repeat the process with another child. Eventually I hand over the leadership to another child in the group who becomes the conductor and eye-pointer. Children will invent their own ways of moving and directing the others and will also often make sure that more than one child is playing at a time.

PURPOSE

This activity is particularly good at assessing children's eye-contact and their general ability to focus and interact in non-verbal ways. Conducting ideas such as this one allow the adults to observe whether the children can take responsibility and lead others, as well as whether they can accept direction and conform. Many children, for example, will be more able to accept direction from another child than from an adult. Sometimes it will also be possible to see whether children can be insightful into each other's needs and whether they can show compassion.

Several different ideas sitting around the large xylophone
DESCRIPTION

I place a large wooden xylophone in the middle of the circle and the children sit around it, near enough to play without having to get up. I explain that we will make a piece of music and that we need to listen rather than talk. I play one note and then hand the beater to the person on my left who plays another note before handing the beater on. Once the beater has gone around the circle we each play two notes, then three, and so on. The challenge may be to reach ten without anyone talking or forgetting what to do.

A variation to this idea could be that each person plays once more than the person before. Another version could be that I play two notes, look at someone in the group who then copies my two notes. That person then plays two of his or her own to be copied by another child, and so on.

Yet another variation is to throw a large dice gently on the xylophone. Whatever note the dice lands on is the note the child starts on. The number on the dice indicates how many notes the child plays. The child then hands the beater to another child who has a turn.

One child could be the leader and hold up one to five fingers to another child indicating how many times the instrument should be struck. Once a conductor has finished, the group gives the child a round of applause and another child has a turn.

If the group is quite settled and the children seem prepared to listen to one another they could all form a slightly larger circle and sit slightly away from the xylophone. One child is invited to improvise on the instrument. When the child has finished playing, the beaters are passed on to another child who then plays in the centre of the circle. Sometimes I might support the improvisations by accompanying quietly on the piano.

PURPOSE

All these ideas involve taking turns and working as a group, allowing us to assess how easy or difficult this is for the children. We can also look at basic number skills and whether children can remember notes that have been played. The last idea also enables us to assess whether children can make their own beginnings and endings.

Group story
DESCRIPTION

In this activity the children are encouraged to think of key words related to a theme and then to choose an instrument to accompany this word. For example, if the theme is Christmas, the word chosen might be reindeer and the instrument a woodblock. Each child will have a key word and an instrument. I sit at the piano and tell an improvised Christmas story while accompanying myself on the piano. Whenever I say any child's key word they play their instrument. When I say the word 'Christmas', the whole group plays together. The children also enjoy telling the story and directing this activity.

PURPOSE

We will be able to assess whether children can make choices and be imaginative, and whether they can listen and follow instructions. We will also be able to see whether they can direct an activity and make up a coherent story, and whether they can negotiate and co-operate within the group.

Guitar conversation
DESCRIPTION

Two children sit back-to-back in the middle of the circle, each holding a guitar. One child has the big guitar and is the question asker, the other child has the small guitar and is the question answerer. Each child asks three questions whilst accompanying himself or herself on the guitar. An answer is given, also accompanied by the guitar. They then swap around and the asker becomes the answerer and vice versa. In this dialogue the guitar becomes the focus of the attention, enabling children who would normally find it difficult to perform to the group to take part.

PURPOSE

These guitar exchanges will allow us to note whether questions can be thought of, what kind of questions they are and how much help, if any, is needed. We can also observe the other children and note how they respond and whether they can listen to the performing duo.

Free choice
DESCRIPTION

The children are sometimes offered a free choice towards the end of the group session. For many children this is a strong incentive to manage the rest of the group. I may refer to the free choice at various points throughout the group to encourage and motivate children to manage their behaviour. Each child chooses an instrument and performs to the rest of the group. Occasionally I might support and accompany a child on the piano but only if this has been requested by the child. Sometimes children choose an electronic keyboard with a built-in rhythm section and will improvise dance music. Some groups of children like to dance and move to this music. This is encouraged only if the performer agrees.

PURPOSE

The children's free choices allow us to see whether children can respect each others' opinions and wishes, listen to each other and express praise as well as receive it. For the performer it is an opportunity to play freely and to be briefly in control of the group. Issues of self-esteem and self-confidence can be observed in this activity. Will a child play at all? How does he play? How long? What is his body language expressing? Is the child uncomfortable at being in the limelight or does he have a need to be in it and cannot tolerate others taking over? Does the child enjoy playing or is he very inhibited?

Playing with the clarinet or the viola
DESCRIPTION

One half of the group sits around the large wooden xylophone while the other half sits around the large metallophone. When I play the clarinet the xylophone group accompanies me; when my viola-playing music therapy student plays her viola the metallophone group plays. We improvise in the same modal key so we can hand the melody over to one another smoothly, and sometimes we incorporate brief silences where everyone is quiet, or moments when we purposely play together and the whole group joins in. This particular idea grew out of having a viola player on placement with me but could be adapted to include any other instrumental player.

PURPOSE

Children will often be moved to hear orchestral instruments played live in front of them and we can observe their emotional responses and their abilities to listen. We can also look at how well they work as teams and whether they are able to maintain interest.

Closing activity
DESCRIPTION

The activity used to bring the session to a close varies. I may involve the children in a discussion and ask each child what his or her favourite and least favourite aspect of the group was. Alternately a goodbye song similar to the 'Hello' song at the beginning of the session may be used. I could also use another imaginative activity involving passing a clap around the circle in cupped hands. On other I might sing a goodbye song incorporating the children's names. Sometimes the children will offer their own ideas as to how the session should end.

PURPOSE

At the end of the session, I aim to bring the group together in a reassuring way. The children who have been experimenting with issues of control will feel safe when I am clearly leading the group again for this closing activity. For some groups it may be useful to bring out and remind the children of important moments in the session.

Another important aspect of the closing activity is that I must say goodbye to the children who are leaving the unit before the next music group. This could be a sensitive issue and might need to be briefly acknowledged without being dwelt on at length. However, in other cases, particularly if a child has been on the unit a long time, it might be important to spend more time thinking about a child's last music group at the Croft. Sometimes I ask the other children to consider what music or musical activities will help them to remember the children who are leaving.

The closing activity can also prepare the children for the next part of their day. If the group has been very active and energetic, for example, I will choose the most appropriate activity to calm everyone down and prepare them for going back to the dining room.

Endings and transitions are difficult moments for many of the children at the Croft. The ways in which the children deal with both the ending of the group and the comings and goings of the children from the unit will be observed and noted.

Reviewing the group

Reviewing the group with the co-worker plays an integral part in the group process. It is an opportunity to share and discuss our observations and decide which key points we want to feed back to the team in the weekly management meetings. As the co-worker works with the children at different times of the day, her opinions are often a very useful and interesting insight into how the music is affecting the children. She will be in a good position to judge whether they are behaving in an expected or unexpected way and whether the musical activities engage children more or less than other interventions on the unit.

Each child will be considered separately and a brief paragraph will be included in the on-going nursing notes, which are written up on a daily basis, in individual files for each child.

It is also important to review how the co-worker and I are working together, and to address any difficulties or tensions in a frank and open way.

Four vignettes

As indicated at the beginning of the chapter, the first three case studies were written by my colleague, Emma Davies. The fourth vignette, Clarissa, was one of my recent cases which I have included to give an example of an older, more adolescent, child in the group.

Carl

Carl was nine years old and was admitted to the Croft because it was felt that he might have an autistic spectrum disorder. He was finding school increasingly difficult to manage, often becoming aggressive and sometimes violent. Teachers observed that he tended to befriend children who were younger than him and did not interact very much with peers of his own age. Carl remained at the Croft for four months, during which time he was a member of the music group as well as having weekly individual music therapy sessions.

In his individual sessions it was clear that Carl enjoyed music making and was able to interact through his playing as long as he felt a degree of control over the structure of the interactions. As sessions progressed his playing became freer and he was more willing to experiment and take risks.

In his first group it was observed that Carl had difficulties in grasping instructions and in accepting that he was not always first or correct in an activity, and he seemed to have little awareness of his peers. When asked to choose an instrument and play freely, he played a pre-composed melody from a television programme. As it was a short melody, the music therapist invited him to play for a little longer. He played the same melody and became quite agitated when he played a part of it incorrectly. However, it was observed that he did participate in all the activities and seemed to have periods of allowing himself to engage in the music.

Carl spent the next few sessions familiarising himself with the structure of the group and getting very involved in the order of events. He would want to explain what each activity involved, both to the adults and his peers. Perhaps he needed to do this in order to feel a sense of control over the situation. Gradually, as he became more familiar with the structure of the group, he began to relax and became more aware of his peers, commenting that it was somebody's turn next or that a particular instrument was being chosen frequently that week. He also began to appreciate the humour of some of the activities and particularly enjoyed it when he thought the music therapist had finished playing a song but then caught children out by continuing to play.

After six sessions it was noticed that Carl was able to cope with the introduction of some new activities. He may have been able to do this because the group had become familiar to him and he was beginning to trust the adults to help with any difficulties he might experience. This was obviously a key point to feed back to the team.

Other insights that were shared with the team were his ability, over time, to accept the fact that he could not always win in a game and that other people may have different opinions and preferences to him but he did not need to change his views. We also discussed his increasing ability to relax, be creative, imaginative and enjoy himself. The co-worker in the group commented that she never found it a problem to bring Carl to the music group, whereas in some other situations he has displayed a certain amount of reluctance. This was important to share with the team as it demonstrated that Carl could manage if he was motivated enough.

For Carl, the rigidity and need for control that he initially showed in the group confirmed the team's suspicions that he was on the autistic spectrum. Nevertheless, his enjoyment of the sessions and his increasing acceptance of his peers showed that when he was sufficiently motivated he could overcome some of his difficulties. In the light of his previous difficulties at school, it was particularly important to establish that, given the right circumstances, this boy could enjoy and interact appropriately with other children of his own age.

Bettie

Bettie was ten years old and was referred to the Croft for a reassessment of her diagnosis of obsessive compulsive disorder (OCD), for a medical trial and for further advice regarding her own management of her difficulties. She attended the unit as a day patient for five weeks. During that time she took part in five group music therapy sessions and four individual music therapy sessions. Staff were interested in how Bettie would interact with her peers in the group and whether she would be able to relax and participate in musical activities.

In group sessions, Bettie initially presented as quiet and tentative. Some of her OCD patterns of behaviour were observed, such as twirling, squinting and requesting that certain notes should not be played. She interacted very little with her peers, except to complain when someone was playing too loudly. Her eye-contact was poor except during a conducting activity when she played the part of conductor in a confident and convincing way, looking at peers and directing their playing. During the last two groups she appeared much more animated, especially during free improvisations, and it was clear that she enjoyed music making. This was particularly interesting as her free and creative playing seemed in direct contrast with the very strict rules she usually placed on herself. On one occasion she had started to refuse to talk but then could not resist joining in and mouthed the words to the 'Hello' song. She has also started a habit of putting her sleeves over her hands, but still persisted in playing, allowing one finger to emerge in order to play the autoharp.

Bettie seemed to find the one-to-one interaction of individual sessions much easier to tolerate than the group setting. She appeared much more relaxed and was able to explore improvisation in a very creative and expressive way. Although there were no playful interactions, and very little eye-contact, Bettie was able to interact musically by initiating her own musical ideas as well as imitating and responding to the therapist's.

In the team's discussions about Bettie in the weekly management meetings, it was important to let the team know that Bettie seemed to find individual sessions more comfortable than group sessions. However, mention was made of the fact that, even when Bettie's OCD behaviours were at their most extreme, she was still able to play and be part of the group. She refused to talk and touch the instruments directly but was still able to be a functioning member of the group. She was able to make choices, participate in most activities or else let the adults know when she did not want to join in.

It is probable that, in addition to Bettie's particular interest in music making, the non-verbal aspect of the group enable her to remain within the session. She also seemed reassured by the predictable structure of the group, which then allowed her the freedom to improvise in a more spontaneous way.

Keith

Keith, who was five years old, was referred to the Croft owing to his increasing difficulties interacting with his peers at school. He was also an elective mute. At home, he would interact normally with his family, but at school he would refuse to talk, walk, sit down, hold anything or eat, and his teachers would have to physically move him from one place to another. His assessment at the Croft was particularly aimed at looking at his interactions with others. Keith remained at the Croft for seven weeks. During his admission he attended the music therapy group as well as weekly individual music therapy sessions.

In individual sessions, Keith was able to make choices of instruments and to play with support. He appeared very engaged during some songs and would look up in anticipation at the end of a phrase, showing an awareness of the song's structure. Bearing in mind that Keith refused to hold anything himself, it was surprising in the second session when he held a violin bow by himself and allowed the therapist to guide his arm to play. During his last week, the team reported that Keith's motivation to communicate seemed to have decreased and the idea that he was expressing anger at having to leave the unit was discussed. In his last individual music therapy session he seemed less motivated to play and did not hold any instruments himself. He also showed less eye-contact. The therapist wondered whether he was using this lack of co-operation to show his discontent at being discharged.

At the beginning of the first group, Keith appeared tense and a little anxious. He refused to sit down and would move only when physically encouraged by a member of staff. Although his posture and body language expressed anxiety and reluctance or inability to participate, his facial expressions showed that he was curious and interested in what was going on around him. He would very slightly turn his head to the source of a sound and would also follow a turn-taking activity with his eyes.

As the sessions progressed, Keith seemed to relax more and, although he still would not sit down or actively involve himself in anything, he began to look expectantly at whatever instrument was going to be played next. During an activity where the children had to guess what instrument was being played behind the piano he could not resist looking around to see what was being played. The adults wondered whether he was making guesses in his head and then checking to see whether he was correct. Mostly he was content to be moved around by staff, but on one occasion he spontaneously moved himself so that he was ready for the activity. Keith also made choices by looking at his preferred instrument. In his fourth session, he chose an instrument and then guided the co-worker's hand to it so that she could play with him. Keith also demonstrated an awareness of the humorous side of activities by smiling and even, on one occasion, trying to restrain a small giggle.

For a child who had such immense difficulties expressing himself and making his needs known, it seemed that the non-verbal aspect of the music therapy group enabled Keith to explore the possibilities of interacting with his peers without having to actually speak or even move. It was very important to feed back to the team that Keith *could* and *did* express some of his feelings of enjoyment and amusement in the group and that he was, on some occasions, able to overcome his restrictions and was motivated to play. He also demonstrated an understanding of verbal and visual instructions and was able to communicate his choices. It was important to feed this back to the team as they were aspects that were unique to the music therapy group.

The co-worker commented that it was the fact that he enjoyed music so much, as well as the security he felt due to the familiarity of the structure, that enabled him to relax and let the adults help him. She also thought that he was able to relax in the music group because he did not feel under pressure to participate, but was allowed to take part in his own unique way.

Clarissa

Clarissa was a 12-year-old school refuser who was presenting behaviour problems both at home and at school. She was admitted to the Croft with her mother to look at her educational needs and assess where she would best be placed in the future, as well as to advise her mother on behaviour management strategies.

Clarissa was seen for eight group music therapy sessions while she was at the Croft. She and her mother were also offered individual music therapy sessions together, but Clarissa refused to come to these.

Initially, Clarissa was reluctant to come in or take part in any way in the group music therapy sessions. In the first session, she brought a book in with her, which she used as a barrier to avoid interaction. On several occasions she would sit on the floor in a corner of the room, listening but not actively taking part. However, she could usually be drawn in to some of the activities and particularly enjoyed drum-playing. She responded well to encouragement and praise and could sometimes be encouraged to take a turn playing in front of the others as long as she did not have to go first.

Clarissa particularly liked quiet, sensitive music played on the clarinet and the viola. On one occasion she played the metallophone with the clarinet and the viola for over ten minutes, appearing to be very engrossed and moved by the mood of the music.

At times Clarissa was quite adolescent and scornful, but at other times she could be supportive of her peers and show a great sense of playful enjoyment. She particularly liked choosing songs for me to play to her on the piano. It often appeared as though Clarissa was happiest when she was able to listen to music or take part in non-verbal interactions where she did not need to talk about what she was doing.

Although it was not easy to engage Clarissa in the music therapy groups, I was encouraged by the fact that this was one of the few groups on the unit that she accepted being part of in any way. I thought that this was probably partly because she could be part of the group by listening rather than having to commit herself to doing anything.

Clarissa seemed very affected by certain types of music, liked listening and occasionally showed an engaging sense of fun and play. My co-worker told me that she felt that Clarissa was showing a sensitive and vulnerable aspect of herself in the music therapy groups that she had not shown at any other times on the unit. Because she was taking part in this group, we were able to report back to the team, in weekly management meetings, that when she wanted she was able to conform to group rules and be caring towards her peers.

In retrospect, I think Clarissa might have been less reluctant to come to individual music therapy sessions if we had invited her to come on her own rather than with her mother. At the time we thought that as she was engaged in the group sessions, family music therapy sessions might be a way of her and her mother having enjoyable moments together. However, Clarissa did not have the confidence to attempt this.

In her discharge report I recommended that, if music therapy were available, I thought she might benefit from longer term individual music therapy sessions where, if she could allow herself to trust the situation, she would have an opportunity to express some feelings and emotions in a non-verbal way.

Conclusion

In this chapter I have described a music therapy group that is used mainly to help the psychiatric team evaluate children's strengths and difficulties. Although this is an unusual purpose for a music therapy group, I feel that this work is immensely helpful to the team at the Croft and a valuable addition to other more conventional methods of assessment.

It is interesting to note that my colleague Emma Davies, who wrote the first three case studies in this chapter, is using the same music therapy approach as I have been describing throughout this book. The musical exchanges are interactive and she is bringing out and focusing on positive aspects of communication. We have worked together for many years and she trained on the music therapy MA course at Anglia Ruskin University.

In the past two chapters I have explored new unconventional ways of using music therapy as an aid to diagnosis. In the next chapter I focus on another relatively new area in music therapy, short-term treatment in child and family psychiatry.

Chapter 4

Individual Short-term Music Therapy in Child and Family Psychiatry

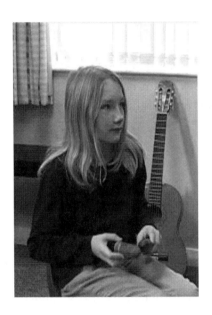

Introduction

Traditionally, music therapy is seen as a slow process that occurs over months if not years. Indeed the Association of Professional Music Therapists (APMT) defines music therapy by saying that it involves 'a relationship between the therapist and client in which music becomes a way of promoting change and growth', (APMT 1997). The development of a relationship in which change and growth can occur clearly presupposes that the work usually goes on for some time. In the late 1990s, as the admissions at the Croft Unit became shorter and shorter, I was forced to re-evaluate my role because traditional long-term music therapy treatment was no longer a possibility. In the previous two chapters I described how I developed individual and group music therapy diagnostic assessments. In this chapter I explore short-term music therapy treatment. I first describe three brief case studies and reflect on this work. I then look at how I worked with a psychotherapist, Christine Franke, to help children through looking at their musical stories. We jointly wrote a chapter about this work for a book about song writing in music therapy, and some of the material from that chapter is used here (Oldfield and Franke 2005).

Other approaches to short-term music therapy

A small number of music therapists have written about successful short-term interventions. Bunt *et al.* (1987) described an eight-week group for adults in the psychiatric unit of a general hospital. Although work with adults is bound to be very different from the approach with children, it is interesting to note that some of the aspects of the work which the authors consider to be unique to music therapy overlap with my views about why music therapy is useful. For example, the fact that both the music therapist and the child are involved in an equal way in the creation of a common musical improvisation, and the fact that the child can do something for fun and enjoyment, are similar.

Edwards (1999b) and Griessmeier (1994) both worked with children in general hospitals. The medical setting was very different from that of a child and family psychiatric unit. Nevertheless, both authors emphasised the importance of working with the hospital team, and the fact that the music therapist must have a very flexible approach. This is certainly similar to the work at the Croft where I often have to change times or approaches at the last minute to fit in with special circumstances. Indeed it could be argued that short-term music therapy has the capacity to be particularly adaptable and varied, lending itself well to children with acute medical and psychiatric needs.

Froehlich (1984) was able to demonstrate that music therapy was more effective than play therapy in facilitating the verbalisation of hospital experiences and feelings. The children in this study had only one-off music therapy and play sessions. Although the client group and the setting were different, it is encouraging to find that results can be obtained from such short-term interventions.

Molyneux described her work at a unit for child and family psychiatry, where a series of fixed-term employment contracts forced her to examine the value of short-term music therapy treatment (Molyneux 2001). She made interesting parallels between short-term music therapy work in child and family psychiatry and Daniel Stern's 'serial brief treatment' (Stern 1995). In both cases, parents and children were treated together and the emphasis was on supporting the mother and creating a positive, non-judgemental environment. She then went on to draw out several points that she felt were features of a short-term approach to music therapy. These were:

- a positive therapeutic alliance
- an active stance of the therapist to engage the client
- containment and structure
- attention to therapeutic aims.

Molyneux trained on the Anglia Ruskin University Music Therapy MA training course and did one of her main clinical placements with me at the Croft. Her work has many points in common with my approach.

All the short-term music therapy described here shows that music therapy can have an important impact, even in a reduced amount of time. There is some evidence that music therapy is particularly well suited to address immediate short-term difficulties and to adapt to unexpected situations.

Four case studies

The following four case studies are examples of children I treated both individually and within the weekly music group at the Croft Unit. Many of the children I work with are seen with their parents or siblings. I shall give examples of the family work in Chapter 5.

Heather

Heather, her mother and her four-year-old sister were admitted to the Croft because Heather was seriously underweight and had been diagnosed with anorexia nervosa. She was ten years old and had been progressively eating and drinking less and less over a period of six months. She had then been admitted to the children's ward at Addenbrooke's Hospital where she was tube-fed and put on bedrest. She was referred to the Croft after two weeks in hospital, once her weight was no longer so low that she needed to be in bed. Her illness had started as a reaction to her parents' very acrimonious divorce.

Heather took part in the daily programme at the Croft with the other children, and weekly special individual counselling sessions as well as family therapy sessions were organised to try to address some of the original reasons for Heather's illness. In addition, Heather was referred to me for individual music therapy sessions to try to help her to be engaged and spontaneous as she was generally very low in mood and completely lacked motivation or enthusiasm to do anything.

During her four-month stay at the Croft I saw Heather for 12 individual music therapy sessions and 14 group music therapy sessions.

INDIVIDUAL SESSIONS

Heather was initially reluctant to come, saying that she was not feeling well and that loud music would give her a headache. I suggested to her that the only music she would listen to would be what she played herself and that we could sit in silence while we decided what to play. As soon as we got to the room she indicated that she wanted to play the piano. I suggested that we should play together and quietly supported her improvisations in the bass on the left side of the piano while she played on the upper right side.

It was immediately apparent that Heather she was very musical and had a good sense of harmonic structure as she managed to play with two hands and found notes in the left hand to accompany her right-hand melodies. She told me that she had had no previous music lessons but that she often experimented on her sister's keyboard at home. Later I was to find out that she had helped her older brother with his GCSE music exam.

In our sessions, Heather would completely immerse herself in her playing and often kept going without looking up from what she was doing for 15 minutes at a time. It was hard for me to support her musically because the rhythms she used were irregular and the melodies seemed to lack direction. She did not seem to be very aware of my playing or react to my musical suggestions. While playing with her I often felt frustrated and lost and wondered whether this was how she was feeling.

When the piano-playing came to a tentative end she allowed me to choose some other instruments for us to play together, but I felt she really would have preferred to continue playing the piano.

After a couple of sessions I suggested that we might record some of her piano compositions, which she agreed to. She listened carefully to her recording and spent time thinking of a suitable title for her piece. From then on we established a pattern where Heather would bring a short composition she had worked on during the week on the keyboard which we would work on together and then record. An important part of this process was always choosing a name for the composition and then listening to the recording. As the weeks progressed Heather would refer back to previous compositions, discussing them and comparing them. Occasionally we would listen to several compositions from different weeks and Heather would usually try to get me to say which one I liked best.

As the weeks progressed, Heather's playing become more rhythmically structured. She would allow me to make suggestions and enjoyed construct-ing pieces using different themes and at times allowing me to play instru-ments such as the xylophone, the metallophone and the conga drums, instead of us both playing the piano all the time.

After her initial reluctance, Heather became openly enthusiastic about our sessions together, often requesting to practise in the music room in the evening. She then started playing her compositions to her mother and to other staff members. She was obviously pleased with the praise she received from everyone about her excellent compositions.

IN GROUP SESSIONS

Heather was initially very shy and quiet and seemed to want to give the impression of being very miserable. I mentioned to her that she looked fed up but that I knew that she had opportunities to talk to staff at the Croft on her own and that perhaps she could use those times to bring anything up that was worrying her. I felt it was important to acknowledge briefly that I noticed that she looked sad but that in this setting I was not going to address that particular difficulty.

By the second group session, although she was still quiet and needed encouragement to speak up and make choices, she was engaged throughout, particularly enjoying playing one of her compositions on her own on the piano in front of the group. Heather never minded taking part in 'young' songs or games and sometimes would put on a 'baby' voice, appearing to want to be 'little'. I thought it was good for her to have opportunities to have fun, be playful and enjoy being a child. Perhaps part of her anorexia was to do with not wanting to grow up and lose her childhood, which she had had with both her parents. By being spontaneous and child-like in these sessions and seeing adults also being playful in this way she could understand, or certainly feel, that certain aspects of playfulness did not have to be lost as she grew up.

Towards the end of each of the sessions Heather would make a point of letting us know that she did not want the session to end, or to leave the room, because this group was just before lunch, to which she was reluctant to go. I felt she wanted to make a point of reminding us all about her difficulties and how much she hated eating. Again I made her aware that I was noticing her distress but could not deal with it in this group. During her final two group music therapy sessions, she was so busy taking part in the final activity that she forgot to make her usual anti-food statements.

At Heather's discharge meeting I suggested that she might benefit from having some private piano lessons where part of the lesson was devoted to composition. I put the family in touch with a piano teacher I knew who I thought would be patient and understanding but who was also a good composer himself.

Music therapy was initially one of the few things Heather wanted to do and was able to show enthusiasm for. She was also able to allow herself to be young and playful in music therapy sessions and realise that this playfulness could persist into adulthood.

Later, her musical achievements gave her confidence and something to be proud of, so she no longer had to continuously focus on her eating problems as her only sense of identity.

Paul

Paul, who was six, had attention deficit hyperactive disorder (ADHD) and behaviour problems. He was admitted to the Croft for six weeks as a day-patient to review his medication and give his parents and his one-to-one support assistant in his school advice on behaviour management.

Paul came to six individual music therapy sessions during his stay at the Croft. In his first week at the Croft we quickly realised that he was not going to manage most of the groups on the unit and would need a special one-to-one programme. In the music therapy group in particular, Paul was completely over-stimulated by all the sounds and instruments and become so excited that he started racing around the room and screaming.

In the individual sessions, Paul generally wanted to be in control, but accepted a structure where we took it in turns to choose what we played. I insisted on this structure even when my choices lasted only a minute or two and his took up most of the session. Paul really loved organising me and telling me what to do, but he also responded very well to the drama and excitement of music making, smiling and enjoying quiet moments as well as energetic playing. At times he would be so involved in the musical exchanges that he would forget that he had to be in control and respond to my musical ideas and suggestions.

Paul asked lots of questions and seemed to want things to be explained to him very carefully. He often appeared anxious that I should take time to listen to what he had to say. I felt that he was desperate for me to hear his point of view, both verbally and musically, and for him to feel that he had some control in what would happen next.

I asked Paul whether he would mind if we videoed his individual music therapy session, so that he could show his mother how he played the different instruments. He was delighted about this idea and enjoyed helping me to set up the camera. He also took great delight in showing the video to his mother and to other staff on the unit. It was particularly important for him to have something positive to focus on as he struggled greatly with many aspects of his behaviour on a daily basis.

I was surprised at how intensely focused this little boy was in the individual music therapy sessions, when on other occasions he appeared unable even to sit down. Perhaps it was because, in addition to his natural love of playful music making, I was able to completely devote myself to his needs, allowing him to be in control of me in a positive way and giving him time to feel heard and listened to.

Andrea

Andrea was 11 years old and was an elective mute although she talked a little to her mother at home. She was attending a small village primary school, which had only three classes. She was managing reasonably well at school with supportive teachers and friends that she had known for seven years. She also posed no problems at home. She was admitted to the Croft for the summer term before she was due to go to secondary school, because both her mother and the school staff were concerned that she would struggle to manage in a large secondary school. Her mother could not come in residentially with her because she was a single mother and had work commitments. However, she agreed to attend sessions at the Croft twice a week in addition to talking to staff at the beginning and the end of the week when she brought and collected Andrea from the unit.

Andrea was referred to me for individual music therapy sessions because it was felt that a non-verbal means of communication would be ideal for her, since she was choosing not to use verbal language. She attended a total of ten weekly individual music therapy sessions with me as well as taking part in ten group music therapy sessions.

In the Croft in general and in the music therapy group, Andrea conformed to what was being asked in a quiet, slightly bored, almost adolescent way, as though what we were suggesting was a little beneath her. Whenever a verbal response from her was required she would either slowly nod, shake her head, shrug her shoulders or vaguely point at somebody or something. When pressed she would make a vague, slow effort to answer non-verbally but never showed much initiative or spontaneity. Her mother was also a bit vague, often missing appointments and not reliably collecting or bringing Andrea to the unit at pre-arranged times.

In individual music therapy sessions, Andrea initially appeared disinterested and bored, but perked up a little when I offered her the drum and the cymbal to play. By the third week I realised that her percussion playing was getting louder and she was becoming more engaged in the playing. By week five her playing was really loud and angry and I was struggling to support and match her playing on the piano. She was not expressing this anger anywhere else on the unit, so we all agreed that I should continue to give her as much chance as possible to express herself on the instruments. The rest of her individual sessions all followed the same pattern. After a brief few chords on the guitar to mark the beginning of the session, she would choose the large percussion instruments and I would play the piano. She would play, mostly very loudly and angrily, for 20 minutes and then I would choose something different for each of us to play for a few minutes before a shared goodbye on the bongo drums.

During our improvising I noticed that, in spite of the fact that the playing was continuously loud and angry, Andrea did gradually listen a little more and accept my musical suggestions. Occasionally I would see her smile, but quickly look away if she thought I had noticed. At the end of the playing she always seemed spent and tired but perhaps a little less tense. During the last few sessions, she agreed to blow some horns in my brief choice after the drumming, and on one occasion she even made some vocal sounds into a kazoo and we managed a brief vocal exchange.

At her discharge meeting, the Croft team reported that although Andrea had not presented the staff with any major problems during her admission, neither she nor her mother seemed motivated to work hard enough to make changes, ask questions or try to understand the difficulties. I was particularly frustrated because I felt that Andrea had made some small changes in the individual music therapy sessions and had begun to take a few risks. I felt that if she could have been offered longer-term work she would definitely have benefited. At least I was able to say something positive about the work we had done and make a suggestion with a hopeful component for the future.

Wayne

Wayne, who was 11, was admitted to the Croft with his mother on a residential basis for eight weeks. He had a previous diagnosis of Asperger's syndrome and had had increasing difficulties at his mainstream primary school, refusing to conform or do what was expected until he was permanently excluded. At home, he was reluctant to do anything except watch videos. During his admission it was hoped that he might be helped to conform somewhat to adult rules, and be more interested and motivated in activities other than watching videos. The Croft also aimed to give advice on future schooling and help his mother with general management strategies.

Wayne was seen for six individual music therapy sessions, and seven group music therapy sessions with his peers.

IN INDIVIDUAL SESSIONS

Wayne initially needed to be persuaded to come to the sessions. On the first occasion when I went to get him he refused to come, saying he did not want to be on his own with me. I think he was unsure of what would happen in the music room and did not trust me enough to risk trying something new. The following week, after he had been to a music group that he had very much enjoyed, he came quite happily and seemed very relaxed. On the next occasion, he was having a very difficult day and was showing reluctance to do anything. He initially said he did not want to come but I managed to entice him into the room by telling him that I might be able to teach him the beginning of the 'Star Wars' theme tune, which I had noticed him reacting positively to in the group session. From then on he was always very happy to come, even reminding me of his individual session times if he thought I might forget.

A large part of each individual session with Wayne became teaching him to play the 'Star Wars' theme on the piano. He was extremely motivated and focused, and worked very hard. He struggled to play by ear and easily forgot where he was in his playing. His fingers were stiff and awkward. However, he was absolutely determined and I encouraged and praised him as much as possible. Eventually he learnt to play the tune in his right hand by learning the names of the notes and following a simple score where I had written the names of the notes under each black dot. I gave him a sheet of paper to practise from and the staff on the unit told me that he used the music room whenever possible to practise. He also spent a lot of his time humming the tune. Once he had mastered the tune in his right hand, I showed him how to add a simple accompaniment with his left hand. In the end he was delighted with his achievement and wanted to play the tune to both staff and children at the unit.

As well as working on the 'Star Wars' theme, we also improvised together, with Wayne on the large percussion instruments and myself on the piano. At the beginning of our sessions Wayne would try to organise our playing by telling me how we should take turns, or what rhythmic structure he wanted to use. As his confidence in his own abilities to make music grew, he was able to be more free and spontaneous in the improvisations. He also started teasing me by suddenly stopping and catching me out, for example, and then inviting me to do the same to him. I always knew when he was tense or worried about something because he would then revert to organising our improvisations rather than allowing them to develop spontaneously.

In the last two individual sessions, Wayne and I enjoyed having kazoo dialogues together. He quickly responded to my mood, entering into funny, angry or sad exchanges with dramatic flair and a great sense of fun. During the second of these dialogues I remember thinking what a huge contrast there was between this engaged, creative, spontaneous and emotional exchange, and his earlier insistence on setting rhythmic rules when we played together.

IN GROUP SESSIONS

Wayne was not hesitant to come in, but as soon as he was in the room he made a point of turning his chair around and facing the corner. We decided to ignore this and just continue in an ordinary way rather than drawing the group's attention to Wayne. Gradually he moved his chair around and came closer and closer to the circle. In this way, in his first group, he mostly listened rather than taking part actively. My co-worker and I felt this was enough for the first group session, but the other children in the group wanted to involve Wayne and enticed him into playing an instrument in the 'eye pointing game' towards the end of the session. Wayne seemed delighted and enjoyed playing. As the weeks progressed Wayne was able to be part of the circle from the beginning and became more and more involved, particularly enjoying conducting and then performing his 'Star Wars' piece to the other children. He also liked choosing songs for me to play on the piano. He would still sometimes suddenly refuse to take turns or actively participate. At these times I commented that I thought he might be trying to remind us that he was 'different' or 'special'. I reminded him that he was special because he had learnt to play a tune on the piano that no other child in the group could play.

Wayne was clearly very motivated to learn to play a favourite tune and felt a great sense of achievement when he had mastered the piece. He gained confidence from performing the piece to other people and was able to be different and special in a positive way. As he relaxed and became more confident he also started enjoying humorous and spontaneous musical exchanges both with me and with the other children. In his discharge meeting I recommended that he might enjoy further piano lessons with a patient teacher who would be prepared to teach him the songs and pieces he wanted to learn, rather than going through a traditional teaching method.

Reflections on the four cases

Most of the reasons why music therapy is effective with this client group are similar to those with other client groups already discussed in this book. However, some aspects are a little different.

- In all of the four cases it was the children interest's in the musical instruments and music making which initially *motivated* them to become engaged. Like other children they all were also held and reassured by the predictable *structure* of the sessions. This was particularly the case for Wayne, whose behaviour could be very chaotic and disorganised outside the individual music therapy sessions.

- The music therapy sessions gave the children a chance to be *playful and humorous*, which children like Heather and Wayne rarely allowed themselves to be.

- All four children, but particularly Andrea, used the sessions to *express feelings and emotions* in non-verbal ways. This possibility is extremely important for many children with psychiatric difficulties who are often struggling with unresolved and strong emotions.

- For Heather and Wayne, the music therapy sessions provided an opportunity to *develop an interest* and compose or learn to play pieces. I feel that this therapeutic teaching is a vital part of my work with those children who express an interest in this area. I try to respond to the child's particular request, encourage him or her, and share my passion for music making. After the children are discharged I try to find specialist music teachers in the area who will continue to nurture the child's enthusiasm for learning and playing music. There is more about therapeutic music teaching in Chapter 1.

- One of the most important things about the sessions for all four children, and for most children with psychiatric needs, is that they were able to have positive experiences, relax and begin to feel good about themselves. Their *confidence and sense of self* developed and improved.

Improvised stories, working in partnership with a psychotherapist

How this work evolved

As described in Chapter 2, I have been using improvised stories both in music therapy diagnostic assessments and in short-term treatment at the Croft Unit for many years. A couple of years ago, the psychotherapist Christine Franke came to observe my work as part of her doctoral research into how children on the autistic spectrum express, process and regulate emotions. We had many discussions about the possible significance of the verbal content of the musical stories. These discussions led to us write a joint book chapter (Oldfield and Franke 2005). The following material is drawn from that chapter.

Description of the musical improvisations

MY MUSIC

I usually start by giving the child a large wooden bass xylophone and a cymbal and sit down at the piano explaining that we will tell a story together. The xylophone was chosen because it is a large, appealing instrument that most children want to try. It is solid but not very loud, so it is possible to hear the song or story at the same time as the instrument is played. The cymbal is usually offered with the wooden xylophone, to allow for loud crashes and a contrasting sound. However, if the child has already used these instruments a lot in other parts of the music therapy session, other instruments such as the metallophone and the drum may be chosen instead.

To begin with, I usually play neutral music to attempt to create a bland and reassuring atmosphere without associations. If the child starts playing immediately my introduction will be influenced by the child's playing: I might match the child's rhythm for example, or pick up on a characteristic short melodic phrase. If the child does not play I might be influenced by his or her posture or expression, or by the style of improvising that has preceded the improvised song. When the child has been offered a diatonic xylophone with no sharps or flats I will usually play in C major, using simple non-confrontative IV(subdominant)–V(dominant)–I(tonic) type chord sequences, in order to fit in with (and not clash with) the child's improvising. At this point I am careful not to play well-known tunes or phrases that might have specific associations for the child. I will sing in a similar musical style, using the words 'Once upon a time, there was a...', pausing in an expectant way after the 'was a...' to encourage an answer from the child.

Some children will immediately play music with me and a musical interlude may then precede the story-telling. Other children will be encouraged to engage by my opening words to the story, and I will then match my accompaniment to the child's playing at the same time as starting the story.

Once the story gets going, my musical accompaniment can either support or interrupt the storyline. I can support the story musically by providing appropriate sound effects, such as: a fast chromatic scale to illustrate running; a sudden two-handed clashing loud chord at the bottom of the piano for a crash; spooky, repeated chromatic phrases to increase tension; or slow, quiet, pentatonic phrases at the top of the keyboard to illustrate peaceful sleep. I may interrupt by suddenly stopping, changing style, inserting a clashing chord, or changing tempo or dynamics. Sometimes I provide longer musical interludes in order to give a child time to think about an issue. Similarly, a verbal phrase in the story may be repeated in a variety of musical ways in order to give particular words value, or to give the child time to think about the sequel.

THE CHILD'S MUSIC

Each child's music is unique, but there are some patterns that seem to emerge regarding the ways in which the children use the music in these stories.

For many children it seems to be the music making that initially draws them into the shared activity and then enables them to create stories and songs. Some children immediately start singing as soon as the therapist sings. Children are often uninhibited musically but more stuck verbally, playing or singing freely but either not speaking at all or producing unconnected words.

Styles of singing will vary, from choirboy voices to rock or rap, from plainsong to operatic-type vibrato or recitative. Sometimes children will 'become' a particular favourite pop singer, or suddenly switch from one style to another. Other children will choose to speak rather than sing.

Many children use patterns in their playing and their singing, either repeated rhythmic patterns such as the 'shave and a toothbrush' rhythm, or short repeated melody lines. Sometimes the children lose themselves in these musical repetitions and forget about the storyline altogether. Occasionally children will become diverted from the storyline by wanting to produce a particular tune or recreate a special sound effect. I can gently attempt to re-engage the child in the story-telling and observe how easy or difficult this might be for the child.

How I guide and support the child's verbal contributions

After the introduction, I might encourage a child to get going by saying or singing 'Was it a dog or a cat? for example. I often suggest familiar domestic animals because many children will be interested in these animals and will easily make associations, which will produce imaginative ideas. Sometimes I might start the story with 'Once upon a time there was a... [and if the child says nothing] ...a boy.' But introducing people rather than animals can more easily lead to an account of something that happened rather than a new story, which is what is being aimed at. If the child starts a well-known story such as 'Once upon a time there were three bears', I might attempt to change things a little by saying something like: '...and they lived in a castle with a magician'. In a similar way children can get stuck in repetitive sequences, so if the therapist feels that there is no more to be gained or learnt from these repetitions, she might purposely interrupt or try to help the child change direction. I could introduce a change by making a new verbal contribution or by making a significant musical change (e.g. a sudden change of volume, rhythm or style).

In many cases, but particularly if the child has not brought any confrontation into the story, I will attempt to incorporate an element of adversity such as a crocodile, a wolf or a monster. This increases the emotional tone of the story and allows me to observe how the child deals with confrontation and possibly help the child to deal with fears or anxieties.

I often choose elements to bring into the stories because of specific previous knowledge of a child's likes and dislikes or particular strengths or difficulties. Many children on the autistic spectrum have favourite topics such as 'aliens' or 'turtles', so I may introduce an alien or a turtle in order to engage and interest a child. Conversely, I may take care to avoid aliens or turtles if I feel these topics will mean that the child becomes isolated in set stories rather than allowing imagination to flow. Other children may be very emotional about their pets, or sensitive about a recent pet's death, so these characters may not be suggested unless I feel it would be useful for the child to use the story to talk about these difficulties.

Often I try to help children to accept my verbal ideas as well as initiate their own, particularly when I feel that a child has begun to take on some of my musical suggestions and seems to enjoy this type of exchange.

If a child brings violence or conflict into a story, I make sure that there is an opportunity to resolve the issues if the child chooses to. However, I will not steer the child towards a resolution, and I will allow him or her to make an unhappy ending if that is what the child wants.

The overall structure of the songs and stories varies completely from one child to another. Some of the children's stories may be no longer than one or two sentences, while others may last 20 minutes and have a clear beginning, middle and end. Apart from the introductory sentence and suggestions to help get things going, I will not seek to guide the structure in any way.

However, I always try to help the children make a clear ending to the story, supporting them to find a way to finish in whatever way is accessible to them. Younger children might say 'one, two, three finish', others might say 'and they lived happily ever after' or simply 'and that's the end of the story'.

Three stories told by Allan, Lee and Thomas
ALLAN'S STORY

Allan was aged 12 and had a diagnosis of autistic spectrum disorder. He was admitted because he was having violent outbursts, had been excluded from school and was struggling at home, often being aggressive towards his mother. He had engaged freely in the musical dialogues with me in the session before the story was suggested. As soon as I started singing 'Once upon a time there was a...' he started playing and singing freely. His singing style matched the diatonic notes he played on the bass xylophone and fitted in with my melody line. He sang about a troll called Albert and a Mummy troll. Albert bought some goggles and they went swimming. At this point I said: 'and suddenly they saw a crocodile…what happened?' Allan continued playing but did not sing or say anything. I encouraged a response by playing unresolved cadences and questioning phrases. Suddenly Allan started chanting an unconnected rap: 'Hey, baby, yea, I'm playing today, one two three, I'm playing today.' I then said 'But what happened to the trolls in the story when the crocodile came?' Exasperated, Allan replied 'The crocodile exploded…and that was the end of the story.'

I was impressed with Allan's creativity and by his ability to listen to my musical ideas as well as initiate his own ideas. I found myself enjoying making music with Allan and felt that he was communicative through his playing. However, he was not willing to incorporate my verbal suggestions into the story. The psychotherapist pointed out that he might have suddenly ended the story because he wanted to avoid thinking about conflicts and be unwilling to explore violence in a story. For the Croft team it was important to find out that Allan could be more communicative in a reciprocal way when he was using a non-verbal form of exchange than when he was talking. This contributed towards the Croft suggestion that he was on the milder end of the autistic spectrum. It was also useful to find out that he was deliberately shying away from talking about violence or aggression, indicating that he was in some way aware of these difficulties in his life, but unwilling to talk or think about them at the moment.

LEE'S STORY

Lee was aged five and diagnosed as having autistic spectrum disorder. His story went like this:

> Once there was a black cow, his name was Lee. (And where did she go?) The farmyard where she met a lady called Lorna Hex. (Lee insists on the 'Hex' being used.) Lee the black cow and Lorna Hex go to the beach and there is a man there and they play with a ball. (I take the story on and continue in an excited tone of voice: As they play the water comes nearer and nearer and what happens?) They drown. (Just like that?) Yea.

I repeat the last part of the story and then ask Lee if we should make an ending. 'Let's count to four.' We do, and end together.

Lee's story is relatively unimaginative. He uses his own name, and although the cow may have some meaning to him this seems not so likely.

The name Lorna Hex seems to be a person he knows and, one imagines, he likes, as he insists on the full name being given. The story is told in early summer, so the beach will probably have been talked about at home or at school. When I take the story over, both musically by energetic and excited playing and also in adding to the story, Lee stops the story: 'They both drown.' It was said in a very definite way. This might indicate that Lee deals with emotional situations by blotting them out rather than confronting them.

The psychotherapist had observed Lee in other settings apart from the improvised story. She was therefore able to note that there was a pattern emerging whereby, whenever he was over-stimulated or the level of emotional arousal was too hard for him to process, he seemed to disconnect from contact. During the story there were times when he fidgeted or appeared to ignore my suggestions. So in this story, the drowning of both the characters is in keeping with the other observations of his dealing with emotional events: there is no thought or processing, just a cessation.

THOMAS' STORY

Thomas was aged seven and had previously had a diagnosis of autistic spectrum disorder. He appeared quite sociable and asked adults many appropriate questions. He obviously thought about what he saw and about what was going on. However, he tended to ignore other children and at times seemed unaware of events happening around him. Thomas had a small alien figure in his pocket and brought it out as he had his session. The alien would do things that Thomas did not want to do, such as hold the beaters. This was his story:

> Once upon a time there was an alien. (Where did the alien go?) He went to the moon. (Who did he meet?) A dinosaur. (And what did they do together?) They made a pie with a cherry on the top. (What was the alien called?) Alfie. (And what is the dinosaur called?) Bailey. They went shopping and then they returned to earth to find something to eat. (And what did they eat?) They ate a doggie's bone. Then they went to the playground and met a spider, who was called Cymbal. (What did they all do?) They had a chat and went together to the seesaw. They all went to the forest and met a tiger and ran away. (I play in an excited manner.) They got away just in time but one was captured – the spider, Cymbal. ('Oh dear', I say.) But they had a plan – they made a monster and the tiger flew away. (Is that the finish?) The spider was saved and they lived happily.

The psychotherapist suggested that this story could have a meaning for him and that the three characters represented aspects of his own self. Thomas may well have identified himself with both the alien and the dinosaur, Bailey. It feels possible that Thomas has a book about a dinosaur and that it was an isolated and perhaps ostracised creature. The creatures were happy in the 'other world' of the moon as they made a pie with a cherry on the top: there is an ideal feel to this world. But this was not enough: they needed more food, so they came back to earth – to the normal shared world of others, to go shopping. What Thomas tells us is that the 'food' here is not as special as the pie with the cherry. It is measly food, 'a doggie's bone', that does not seem very good to him.

The psychotherapist imagines that this is how it may feel to Thomas: He wants to be part of the normal world but finds that his autistic world is more fulfilling, it is less stressful and he can withdraw into it. They meet a spider called Cymbal, named after the object in front of his eyes. The psychotherapist felt that this represented the part of himself that is vulnerable when he is on earth. The tiger may represent one of two aspects. It may be the hostile feelings of others that he feels threatened by, and that he uses his alien and dinosaur aspects to rescue his spider self. This could be a happy ending of the three characters reunited, but it suggests there could possibly be a return to the ideal world – that is into an autistic withdrawal. Or the tiger could represent the more protecting defensive part of himself that looks after his vulnerability when he is 'on earth' and keeps the difficult things away. However, the sad part of this is that the 'autism triad' seems to regroup, thus suggesting, again, Thomas' pull to an autistic state.

When feeding back to the team it was important to share that Thomas was thinking about his different worlds and at times consciously retreating into autistic behaviours.

Why these improvised musical stories are useful

Although spontaneous story-telling could be assessed without the improvised music making, the instrument-playing and singing will often motivate a child and fuel his or her imagination. Acting out the story on the instruments makes the story more exciting, and I can improvise on the piano to underline or contain emotions such as excitement, fear or happiness.

The fact that music happens in time and musical phrases can be organised to have predictable lengths with endings that can be anticipated will reassure children and enable some children to relax sufficiently to allow creativity.

Through improvised music making the child and I can be equals as we are both making music freely without reference to a coded language which I may be more at ease with than the child. Some children, however, will not choose to be equal and will really enjoy the fact that they can control me through the improvised songs or stories. I can support and echo these children's stories, giving the child the sense of being listened to and heard. For children who struggle to make decisions and speak up for themselves, I can provide the basic storyline, perhaps limiting the child's decisions to a choice of two items. For the hesitant child, I can provide musical padding to give time for thought processing and decision making. For the impulsive, fast child, the musical accompaniment can be limited to the odd supportive chord.

The playful aspect of the musical interaction will also appeal to many children who may react to dramatic interchange rather than to verbal exchanges.

The particular value of these songs and stories is that they allow me to evaluate how a child interacts verbally as well as non-verbally. A large part of my work focuses on non-verbal musical reactions, so in the improvised songs and stories the way the child uses (or fails to use) words or vocalisations will reveal new information. A child who is relaxed and at ease with me musically may also choose to talk to me and share important feelings in these stories.

Sometimes it is not so much the words themselves that are interesting as the relationship between the words and the music making. The way in which a child switches from verbal to non-verbal types of communication might be particularly striking, or the discrepancy between a child's ability to communicate non-verbally and his or her ability to communicate through language could be significant.

Conclusion

In this chapter I have focused on short-term individual work in child and family psychiatry. I have described a number of very different cases and then focused on the specific use of musical improvised stories. In the next chapter I shall describe work where the child and the parent are both present.

Chapter 5

Music Therapy with Families at the Croft Unit

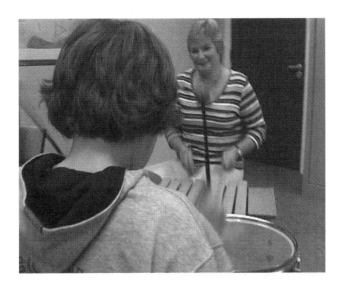

Introduction

In this chapter, I shall describe various types of family music therapy at the Croft Unit. First I look at three different pieces of individual work, then at two types of groups I have run with families. I have written about some of the group work before and will be using material from two earlier articles (Oldfield 1993b; Oldfield and Bunce 2001).

Other family music therapy work

There do not appear to be many music therapists who have written about clinical music therapy with families. Lenz (1996) worked as a music therapist with mothers and young babies who were experiencing excessive feeding and sleeping problems. She believed that these problems were a result of faulty interactions between mothers and babies. She used music therapy techniques to repair the relationships and alleviate the babies' difficulties.

Another music therapist who has worked with mothers and babies is Nocker-Ribaupierre (1999). Her work has been specifically with premature babies and has included playing recordings of the mother's voice to the baby. She felt that it was particularly important for the infant's development to hear the mother's voice in order to have a 'continuum for primary acoustical representation'.

Levinge (1993) described a project with three separate mothers and their young children, concluding: 'music therapy had been able to provide a nurturing facilitating environment in which each couple could be nurtured'.

Bunt (2002, p.73) wrote a case study about two years of individual music therapy with a three-year-old girl with autism and her mother. Many of the themes that the little girl's mother commented on, such as her daughter's need for control and her growing enjoyment in sharing and turn-taking, were similar to those that came up in the semi-structured interviews with the parents in my child development centre outcome study (Oldfield 2006). He concluded this case study by saying: 'The music clearly helped to deepen the relationship between the mother and the child. This was demonstrated particularly in the way Suzanna included her mother in the musical play'.

All these descriptive examples seem to indicate that both parents and children benefit from joint music therapy sessions. Indeed in some cases the families' difficulties can be addressed only when the therapist focuses on the relationship between the parent and the child.

Warwick (1988) concluded an article in which she was describing her work with mothers and young children with autism by saying: 'There is a real need for therapy in the family setting...mothers should have the opportunity to share such a creative experience in sounds and silence, time and space', (p.7). In Warwick's (1995) research into this work, one of the hypotheses investigated was that 'the mother's perception of and attitude towards her child will become more positive'. Results from this project were encouraging.

Thus, although there is not a great deal of literature on music therapy with families, the above texts indicate that music therapy has been successfully used with a wide variety of mothers and children. Music therapy seems to enhance the bond between the parent and the child, enables parents to gain new insights about their relationships with their children, and in many cases improves the quality of life for the child and the parent.

Three families receiving individual music therapy treatment

Nathan and Maya

Nathan was six years old, had mild learning difficulties and was admitted to the Croft Unit because his mother struggled with his difficult behaviour at home. His mother also wanted the Croft to assess whether he was on the autistic spectrum and had attention deficit disorder. Before coming to the Croft he attended a mainstream primary school where he was often excluded from the classroom because he would ignore adults' requests. Nathan was a single child and his father had left Maya before the birth. Maya had never worked and, since Nathan's birth, had suffered from bouts of depression for which she had received medication.

Nathan was at the Croft on a residential basis with his mother for eight weeks. During that time he was seen for six individual music therapy sessions with his mother, two individual music therapy diagnostic assessments on his own and eight group music therapy sessions.

In all of the sessions it was quickly apparent that Nathan loved music making. He particularly liked improvising songs on the guitar, standing up and moving in rock star fashion and imagining that he was playing in a band to a large audience. He would lose himself in his playing and happily invent one song after another, never wanting to finish. He could wait and listen to others if he knew that he would eventually have another turn at playing and performing, but would easily lose interest if he was not playing himself and sometimes even leave the room. He loved directing or conducting other children or adults, but would find it difficult to remain interested in following other children when they were directing.

He showed an excellent sense of rhythm and phrasing, could sing well and recognised a wide range of children's songs. In our musical stories, he would lose himself in the playing and improvising. When asked to contribute to the storyline, he would say the first words that came into his head, often using words with musically interesting sounds or syllables. He seemed to want to choose words with sounds that fitted in with the music, but was oblivious to the fact that the words did not make sense in the story. When I tried to help him to follow some kind of storyline, his thinking in these stories seemed to be quite black and white with children being good or naughty and characters being dead or alive.

In the sessions with Nathan and his mother, I would sing 'Hello' on the guitar and then we would each take turns choosing instruments for all three of us to play together. When it came to my turn I would sometimes suggest that we should take it in turns to lead or conduct the other two. At other times I suggested ideas like the counting games on the xylophone described in Chapter 3. Afterwards Maya and I would discuss the session together while Nathan went to join the other children. Sometimes we videoed the sessions and looked at videos of previous sessions to guide our reviews.

Nathan was very attached to his mother and was delighted when they came to music therapy sessions together. He seemed desperate to please her and gain her approval. Maya's attitude to Nathan varied tremendously depending on her own mood. In some sessions she would be quite critical of Nathan, and seemed to pick up on the things he could not do and was keen to point out all his inadequacies to me. I even thought that she sometimes set him up to fail, giving him instruments she knew he would not like and choosing instruments to play herself that she knew he particularly wanted. There were occasions when Maya's criticism of Nathan would lead to the two of them being locked in confrontations, with both of them trying to be in control, and Maya would then turn to me and say 'You see this is what he's like at home, all the time.' Nathan would react by being more confrontational towards his mother and they could easily both become stuck in escalating battles. Nathan was very aware of his mother's emotions and clearly was concerned when his mother was cross or upset. On several occasions he told us that he was pleased that his mother was happy, and he would often go up to his mother and give her a hug.

At other times she could not help admiring his guitar songs and performances and would tell me that he was obviously good at music because it ran in the family; she was good at music too. She herself would enjoy playing the instruments and seemed to want to have fun and make music. At times I felt she was desperate to play the instruments herself, almost competing with Nathan for my attention and admiration. She had not had a happy childhood and had never had opportunities to be playful with her own parents. I felt she was using the sessions to catch up on playing in ways she had not had opportunities to do as a child, in addition to discovering how to relax and be playful with Nathan.

In our reviews of the sessions, Maya was often quite negative about Nathan, telling me that he was difficult and naughty. I used the videos of our sessions to try to help her to see the positive sides of his playing and point out that his difficulties with concentration were due to his general learning difficulties and not because he was being naughty. I also focused on how creative Maya herself was in the music therapy sessions. As she relaxed and gained confidence she began to enjoy making music with Nathan and took pride in his obvious musical strengths. It was only towards the end of our six sessions together that Maya started acknowledging that her mood could have an effect on Nathan and sometimes cause him to be sad or happy. I also pointed out to her that many aspects of her mothering had been very positive since Nathan was obviously warm and caring and very attached to his mother.

After four weeks at the Croft the psychiatrist met Maya to report back to her that, although Nathan was obviously not an easy child and was at times very difficult to look after, the team did not feel that Nathan was on the autistic spectrum or that he had an attention deficit disorder. Maya was initially very upset and cross after this meeting because she had hoped that we would find out what was wrong with Nathan and then be able to give advice and medication to put it right. Nevertheless, during the second half of the admission, we were able to help her both to have more realistic expectations regarding Nathan's abilities and to acknowledge that her mood and emotional affect could be influencing the way he was behaving. She also began to feel more positive about her own abilities to manage and to believe that there were things she could change in the way she interacted with Nathan to make their lives easier.

Nathan and Maya were very keen to take a copy of the video of their music therapy sessions when they left. They were both proud of the improvised musical interactions they had had together and wanted to be able to look back at them.

Helen and Linda

Helen and her mother, Linda, were admitted to the Croft on a residential basis for eight weeks. Helen was 12 years old, had Asperger's syndrome and had completely taken control of her mother. She would go to school only when she chose to, would decide what television programmes should be watched, what food should be eaten in the house and which people were allowed to visit. If her mother tried to go against her daughter's wishes, Helen would shout, scream, throw objects about and sometimes even physically attack her mother. Helen's father also had Asperger's syndrome and was supportive of both his wife and his daughter. However, he worked very long hours as a computer programmer and if he met with conflicts when he arrived home he tended to withdraw, leaving Linda to cope.

Linda was very anxious about her daughter, desperate to help, but totally lacking confidence. She was embarrassed and hurt by the way her daughter treated her. She felt she had failed and did not know what to do next.

Helen took part in seven group music therapy sessions with the other children on the unit and six individual music therapy sessions with her mother.

In the group sessions, Helen was able to take part when she had a clear role such as conducting the other children, choosing instruments for each of the children in the group, performing an improvised piece or putting her instrument down very quietly while we all listened. During group playing, or at times when there was less structure, Helen would quickly become restless and silly, making adolescent-type comments about the songs or the music being 'boring'. However, I did not think she really was bored, more that she was anxious about not knowing exactly what was going to happen next and wanted to take control of the situation so that she knew what would happen next.

When she was enjoying herself, performing in front of the other children, Helen showed humour and a great sense of fun. However, she would often be impatient and critical of others, sometimes making unkind or insensitive remarks.

In the sessions with her mother, Helen initially needed encouragement to come and was quite rude and disparaging about doing music with her mother.

As in the previous case, in general, we all three took turns to choose what we would do. However, after a quick 'Hello' where we each played the bongo drums in turn, I started every session by giving both Helen and Linda the largest and loudest percussion instruments in the room, and encouraging them to play as loudly as they wanted while I supported the improvisation on the piano. Both Helen and Linda would play very loudly for up to ten minutes, sometimes shouting and vocalising at the same time. This seemed to release tension and give both Helen and Linda a chance to let go. Helen seemed to enjoy being part of the controlled chaos and was stimulated and excited by the loud sounds. She was both incredulous and pleased that both her mother and I were joining in what appeared to her to be 'wild' and 'cool' playing. Linda appeared to use this playing as a way of expressing frustration and anger in a constructive way. The loud playing also drowned out any of Helen's unpleasant comments to her mother. I felt Linda's playing had a desperate as well as very angry feel to it, which was in stark contrast to her usual apologetic and self-conscious attitude; she was always very polite and positive, as well as being almost embarrassingly grateful for anything I might suggest or do.

After this very loud and cathartic playing, Helen was usually more able to accept her mother's and my musical suggestions, as well as taking great satisfaction from the fact that we would pick up on her musical ideas. In our musical dialogues it was possible to make indirect suggestions to Helen and enable her to somewhat relinquish the overwhelming control she was exerting over her mother. Linda would feel strengthened both by releasing anger and by being listened to, and would then be more prepared to stand up to Helen when necessary.

In the fourth of our sessions together, I suggested that the three of us should play kazoos. A very lively vocal exchange quickly evolved with both Helen and Linda enjoying the humorous side of the dialogues. I inserted some angry sounds into the trio and Helen quickly entered into playful roaring sounds directed at her mother. Linda responded by roaring back at Helen, remaining playful but nevertheless standing up to and responding to Helen in a far more outspoken and clear way than she had ever done verbally.

As Helen relaxed her overwhelming need to be in control, she consented to perform a pop song to the two of us with great flair and musicality. We applauded, Helen was embarrassed but pleased, and Linda was delighted as, although Helen spent a lot of time on her own in her room singing pop songs at the top of her voice, she had never before consented to perform to her mother.

At Helen's discharge meeting, Linda was very enthusiastic about the music therapy sessions she had had with her daughter. She said that she felt that the musical interactions had given her a chance to have some very positive times with her daughter and had enabled her to feel more confident about her relationship with her. She was hoping to arrange for further private individual music therapy sessions for the two of them in the future.

Oliver, Abigail and Tim

Oliver, who was nine years old, was admitted to the Croft as a day-patient for a period of six weeks. His parents reported that his behaviour was impossible to manage at home and they wanted to have him assessed for attention deficit disorder. At school, teachers reported that he often pushed boundaries and was quite difficult, but that he was bright and able, and could respond to firm, clear boundaries. Oliver had one sister who was two years older and a brother who was three years younger. Neither his sister nor his brother caused any problems at home.

During his six weeks at the Croft, Oliver had two music therapy diagnostic assessments and four music therapy sessions with his parents, and he took part in six group music therapy sessions with the other children.

After the first two weeks the Croft team felt that Oliver did not have an attention deficit disorder but that he was struggling to relate to his parents and anxious about his place within the family. He appeared needy emotionally and greatly lacked self-confidence. However, in music therapy sessions, Oliver presented a very different picture. He had had classical guitar lessons since the age of six and had recently successfully taken his Grade 4. He was obviously an accomplished musician who could read music and also strum chords and accompany singing. In this one area he felt strong and confident and with a little encouragement would perform to his peers who were clearly impressed with his ability.

Oliver's parents, Abigail and Tim, were quite angry when the Croft fed back to them that they did not think he had an attention deficit disorder, but indicated that some family work for the three of them might be helpful to try to improve their relationships. Neither Abigail nor Tim felt that there was anything wrong with their relationship with Oliver. They were convinced there was something wrong with Oliver himself and that if we could only find out what it was he could be given treatment and all would be resolved. In general, they were very negative about Oliver, saying that he was ruining their life and that the other children were suffering because of Oliver's difficult behaviours. However, they were proud of his musical achievements and it transpired that Tim and Oliver often played together, with Tim accompanying his guitar pieces on the piano. It was therefore suggested that they all three take part in four family music therapy sessions with a view to having some positive times together.

In the first two sessions they presented as the perfect family. Oliver and Tim performed some beautiful classical duets to Abigail and myself and we clapped and praised them. In our free improvised musical exchanges everyone played and listened to one another in very supportive and creative ways. When reviewing the sessions with the parents at the end of the session after Oliver had joined the other children, I commented that these very positive musical exchanges they were having together as a family must make up a little bit for the difficulties they experienced at other times. I tried to help them to see how well they had done in enabling Oliver to develop his musical skills, how gifted and able he was, and what a privilege it was for Tim to be able to make music with his son.

In our third session together, I took a slightly different approach. After another very enjoyable guitar and piano duet between Tim and Oliver I suggested that we all four play together, with Oliver leading from the drum, Abigail playing the tambourine, Tim playing the large wooden xylophone and me on the piano. I added that we would be following Oliver's music but that if he wanted he could at times make it challenging for us to follow him. At first the playing started off as before, everyone following Oliver's lead in interactive and creative ways. Then he suddenly stopped, catching all of us by surprise. He laughed when we were unable to follow his increasingly difficult and unpredictable rhythms, delighting in the control he had over all of us. Our improvisation continued for over five minutes at which point I began to give musical indications (for example: gradually slowing down, and clear cadences) that we might bring the piece to an end. Oliver picked up my cues and brought the piece to an end. Tim, however, then added a beat on the xylophone. Oliver responded to this by playing again and we all followed him and our piece continued. I tried again, Oliver responded, we finished together and Tim again had the last word. After about ten false endings, I commented to Abigail, who had put her tambourine down in a cross way after the third ending, that it appeared that father and son were locked in some kind of power struggle. She sighed and said that this was what it was like all the time at home and that her way of dealing with them was to opt out and let them fight it out. Oliver and Tim agreed with her, and Oliver added: 'one of us always has to win'.

In the following and final session all three of them wanted to talk as well as play. We explored both positive and negative sides of Oliver and Tim's musical relationship and started thinking about how the musical and other exchanges did not necessarily need to be 'won' or 'lost'.

At Oliver's discharge meeting I suggested that the family might benefit from long-term family therapy sessions. Although Abigail and Tim had refused to consider this possibility two weeks previously they now were prepared to think about family issues in a more open way.

Reflections on this work

- With these three very different families, issues of *control* were central to all the work. Maya felt cross and frustrated when she felt Nathan was being naughty and out of control. Linda had to work hard to regain at least some control over Helen, and it was a power struggle between Oliver and Tim that seemed to be central to their difficulties.

- All three families also gained great joy and satisfaction from *interacting non-verbally* through music making. The first two families discovered how to do this while they were at the Croft, whereas for the third family it was the one positive experience they felt they were having with their son. The non-verbal aspect of the music therapy sessions was also important for the second and third families because using language was difficult. Helen was verbally abusive to her mother; and Abigail and Tim had initially reacted negatively to any kind of talking therapy.

- All three children loved music making and were very *motivated* to come to the sessions. Tim, Oliver's father, had a particular interest in music making before he came, but for the other adults it was the children's enthusiasm for the instruments that introduced them to the idea of playing.

- For all three families music therapy in some way provided an island of pleasure, a *positive experience* when most of their lives and interactions consisted of struggles and battles. Maya found it helpful to take a video of the music therapy sessions with Nathan home with her, to remind her of the positive moments she had had with her son.

- For Linda, it was particularly important to use loud improvisations to *express her feelings* of frustration and anger. For Maya, the music therapy sessions allowed her to be *playful*, which she had not had many opportunities to do as a child.

- The music therapy sessions enabled all three families to *gain new insights* in to aspects of their relationships. Maya was eventually able to acknowledge that Nathan's behaviour could be affected by her own mood. Linda realised that she had the capacity to be more in control of Helen, and Helen, for the first time, saw her mother as somebody who could be forthright, play loudly and express emotions. Abigail and Tim began to acknowledge that there were issues in their relationship with Oliver that could be discussed and explored, which and might be contributing to some of his difficulties.

A six-week group with mothers* and young children

The six-week music therapy group with mothers and young children was part of a 12-week package of treatment offered by the Croft Unit to a group of mothers and young children, for one morning once a week.

The general treatment package

The aim of this treatment package, which was called the Mother and Toddler Group (MTG), was to help families who were experiencing difficulties in the parenting of their young children. In many cases mothers needed support and encouragement as they had lost confidence in their own abilities as parents. Many mothers who had not experienced good parenting themselves needed to be shown good models of childcare. Some mothers needed help with managing daytime routines, others with how to cope with sibling rivalry. Sometimes there were more specific difficulties. A mother might have been struggling to bond with a particular child, for example, or might have been over-protective and needed help to separate from a child. In addition, it was hoped that by helping mothers of young children in this way, repeated cycles of bad parenting could be changed, making it easier for future generations to enjoy their own families.

Families were referred because their children had extremes of 'normal' behaviour, such as temper tantrums, poor sleeping, eating difficulties, oppositional behaviour, bed-wetting or sibling rivalry. Generally speaking the children had global difficulties, rather than a specific problem. They were initially referred to the outpatient clinic by health visitors, GPs, nursery schools and playgroups. The outpatient clinic then referred families to the MTG, which was run at the Croft Children's Unit.

A member of staff involved with the treatment package would make one or more home visits to a family before that family began to attend the MTG. The visits would serve as an informal assessment and provide an opportunity both to inform the mother about the group and to discuss any fears she might have about the treatment.

---

*   For simplicity's sake, I have used the word 'mother' when referring to the primary carer of the child. In some cases the primary carer might have been the father, another relative, or an unrelated person.

The staff team included an occupational therapist, a community psychiatric nurse, a health visitor, a counsellor and a music therapist. Students and senior registrars frequently joined this team.

The MTG consisted of a weekly two-hour session, running for 12 weeks. The timetabling of the two hours was the following:

9.45 – 10.00	Arrive
10.00 – 11.00	Parents' support group
10.00 – 11.00	Children's playgroup
11.00 – 11.15	Coffee break for mothers, plus staff review
11.15 – 11.45	Weeks 1 to 6: play session; weeks 7 to 12: music therapy session
11.45 – 12.00	Review with families and staff

Even before I was available to work with this group, the nursery nurses employed at the Croft often used music as part of their work with parents and young children, particularly singing songs as a way of rounding off the play session. When I joined the team, the music sessions took on an identity of their own and it was found that parents found it easier to begin with the familiarity of play, rather than the slightly more unusual music therapy. This is why the treatment package included play sessions for the first six weeks, which were then replaced by music therapy sessions for the following six weeks.

Music therapy with the MTG
The following structure describes a typical music therapy session with parents and children. This structure is flexible and may change according to various needs within the group. Sessions usually last about half an hour, which is followed by a 15-minute review with the parents, while the children play with a member of staff in another room. As well as the parents, the children and myself, there is normally another member of staff present in the session.

THE INTRODUCTION

Before starting, a brief explanation of the session is given. I explain that everyone will make music together and that this will help the adults to play with the children. This reassurance goes a little way to put parents at their ease as some may have come with fears about music and performing. The parents are also informed about the number and length of sessions.

GREETING SONG

The beginning of the music therapy session is marked by a quiet greeting song on the guitar which can quickly involve children and parents in strumming the strings of the guitar when their name is sung. Even very young babies can be captivated by live singing and guitar-playing. This fascination frequently gives insecure adolescent mothers the excuse to take part rather than reject what is being offered. This may develop so that the children can choose who is said 'hello' to next. From this initial song we can observe how the families interact, whether they can accept and give direction and whether they can listen to one another.

USING THE INSTRUMENTS TOGETHER

I put a selection of small percussion instruments on the floor for both parents and children to choose and play. I usually accompany the spontaneous playing from the piano, providing a structure for the group to start and stop playing the instruments. The freedom and flexibility of the structure of this activity invariably brings up the issue of how much parents should control and direct their children, and how much they should allow the children to roam freely. Extremes of this behaviour are sometimes seen, where one parent will allow a child to climb on the window sill, whereas another parent will hold on to the child, preventing him or her from choosing an instrument.

FOLLOWING A CONDUCTOR OR MOTHER AND TODDLER SOLOS

Often leaders will emerge out of the group improvisation. I will suggest that a toddler should conduct the group from a large instrument, such as a drum. Many children are delighted by the sense of power that leading a group brings, and parents can enjoy the positive side of their child being in control. This is useful for encouraging listening and giving praise, as each soloist can be rewarded by a round of applause and personal congratulations.

ACTION SONGS

It is useful at some stage in the session to suggest an activity involving movement. This could mean encouraging parents and children to do 'Row, Row, Row Your Boat' type activities, or it could mean dancing, marching, or running round the room. Another example could be parents lifting their children up in the air and pretending they are aeroplanes or jumping frogs. Children with concentration difficulties will be helped by the variety provided by an activity involving movement, and most children will enjoy interacting physically with their parents.

THE ENDING

Sessions have a clear ending, which is in a quiet, relaxing mode, encouraging physical closeness between parents and children. Parents who feel distant from their children will be frequently surprised that they can be relaxed and at ease, rocking to a lullaby with their child. It may be appropriate to take turns to say goodbye on an instrument, or sing songs chosen by the children. It is helpful if the last part of the session is unthreatening and as positive as possible.

Reviewing the session with the parents

After the session is over the children go into a different room with a member of staff while the parents and I review the session. In the review of the very first session it is explained to the parents that the purpose of the session is to address some of the difficulties that the family has been experiencing. It is stressed that the parents are responsible for their children in the session and should praise or direct their children appropriately.

It is helpful to focus on one or two areas of difficulty, such as controlling aggressive behaviour, giving the children more praise, allowing themselves to relax and improvise with their children or dividing attention between siblings. Parents often want to use the review time to talk about their children's problems in other settings, but it is useful to try to help the parents focus primarily on what has just occurred, and how the next session might be approached.

The music therapy session will allow parents to interact with their children in more positive and spontaneous ways than usual. However, it is often only through discussion after the session or by looking at videotapes of themselves in the sessions that parents can recognise that there are times when they can enjoy being with their children. This recognition can raise their hopes and confidence. This in turn provides a starting point for looking at ways of strengthening or improving their relationship with their children.

Music can help recreate a warm, simple interaction between a parent and a child. This may be partly because a mother will remember similar interactions between herself and her own mother. Playing simple musical instruments can help parents to be children again themselves and to rediscover the fun and spontaneity of being a child. This will bring parents closer to their children and they will be able to take part at the same level. The structured, non-verbal nature of many musical activities or improvisations can be very reassuring for families who have become entangled in verbal conflicts, and the delicate issues of control can be redressed. Above all, relationships that have become mainly negative can again be seen in a more positive light, as families rediscover the ability to have fun together through music making.

It is interesting to briefly reflect on the particular role music therapy plays in the MTG and why music has always been part of the treatment programme. Initially, the nursery nurses ended the morning by singing familiar children's songs or action songs. This is a usual activity in pre-school groups and most nursery nurses are taught a wide repertoire of such songs as part of their training. But why are these songs used and what is special about this activity? Young children quickly recognise familiar tunes, and singing well-known songs will be both reassuring and enjoyable. If the songs are always sung at the same time, children will soon associate the song with the ending of the group, for example, and come to expect this usual ending ritual. Unlike other activities such as drawing or putting puzzles together, singing is something all the children do together at the same time, creating a group feeling where all the children are jointly attending. The only other common activity where nursery children attend as a group in this way is story time. But when the teacher is reading or telling a story, the adult has a different role from the children, whereas when singing the adult and the children are all equal.

It can be very helpful for parents and children who are experiencing difficulties in their relationships to be equal in this way. The fact that many musical activities enable young children to function as a group means that skills such as listening to others, waiting and sharing can easily be addressed. Parents will often be surprised at how well their unco-operative toddlers concentrate and listen and may begin to see their children in a more positive light. Music therapy groups are also ideal settings to give children opportunities to perform to others. Childrens' and parents' confidence can be boosted in this way. In addition, children or parents can direct and be in control of music making in the group. This can give parents a chance to see children who they feel are controlling them in a negative way (by being in constant need of adult attention, for example) direct and be in control of the group in a positive way. Mothers might also welcome an excuse to enjoy singing and being playful themselves, particularly if they have never had many opportunities to enjoy playing as children.

Vignette: Tony, Bob and Laura

Tony, aged three-and-a-half years, Bob, aged 20 months, and their mother Laura were referred to the MTG because Laura had suffered from postnatal depression after the births of both of the children. At the time of admission, Laura's mood appeared to have lifted somewhat, but she had days when she felt quite low, lacked confidence and struggled to believe in herself as a good mother.

In the group play sessions, Laura worked hard to involve her children and was loving and caring towards them. However, she lacked spontaneity and did not seem to have much fun herself. She was generally quiet and did not socialise very much with the other families. Tony, however, was quite outgoing and often played with the other children. The other mothers clearly liked him because he was friendly and caring towards the children in the group. At the end of the play sessions, it was fed back to Laura what a popular boy Tony was, and this obviously pleased her.

In the group music therapy sessions, Laura was again quiet at first, even though Tony and Bob immediately took to the instruments and played with enthusiasm and excitement. In the second session the children took turns having solos with their mothers in the middle of the circle. I supported the solos from the piano and when the piece was over everyone clapped. Tony chose the large bass xylophone for the three of them to play together. Laura was soon drawn into the playing and seemed to become more animated than usual, reacting to Tony's energetic musical suggestions. She looked genuinely pleased when the group applauded after the playing. After the session, the other mothers commented on how good Tony and Laura's playing had been. Laura told us that she had always been good at music at school but that her parents had not wanted her to have instrumental lessons. She confessed to us that she had always longed to learn to play the trumpet.

The following week I choose three reed horns for Tony, Bob and Laura to play during their solo. As I gave them the instruments I said to Laura that I was sorry that I did not have any trumpets to offer them, but that at least the reed horns looked vaguely like trumpets. They started to play and the sounds were so loud that Laura pretended to hold her ears when Tony played. He giggled and then started teasing his mother by playing right in her ear. A playful and humorous exchange developed where, in between giggles, Laura, Bob and Tony tried to play loudly in each other's ears. This was the first time we had seen Laura letting go, laughing and having so much fun. At the end of this session, one of the other mothers said that she had an old cornet in her cupboard that she could lend Laura, because her older son no longer played it. From then on Laura brought her cornet to the group and impressed us all as she learnt to play more and more notes. Tony and Bob were obviously pleased with the attention their usually shy and retiring mother was getting from the rest of the group. Laura became more confident and spontaneous as the weeks progressed and above all seemed to have a 'spark' that had not been apparent previously.

One-off interventions followed by video reviews with groups of mothers and babies

These interventions were part of the Parenting Project (PP) which was another weekly outpatient group run by the Croft Unit.

General description of the PP

The PP was different from the MTG in that it was an on-going group for parents with younger children and babies. The project offered individual counselling, a parent/child interaction group aimed at ensuring successful bonding between parent and child, and a support group for parents to address personal issues and concerns. The process was seen as joint work between the families and staff. Hilary Ford (community psychiatric nurse) wrote that many of the parents on the project experienced a difficult childhood where they themselves were inadequately nurtured. This was one of the main causes of difficulties when they became parents. The project aimed to provide the missing ingredients for the parents so that they felt more able to parent their own children effectively (Ford 1994).

Referrals came directly from health visitors, adult psychiatric services, social services, GPs or the parents themselves. Reasons for referrals included: postnatal depression; other past or present mental health problems on the part of the parent; parents who were themselves victims of abuse; or parents who had had difficulties parenting previous children. Generally the participants in the project were women. The majority of these women were either single parents or, in many cases, had an unsupportive partner.

Before and during the project potential families were visited at home by a member of the team for an informal assessment. This was an opportunity to gather background information about the family and assess what specific issues might have been presenting as a problem. Several home visits were sometimes necessary to build up a parent's confidence, so that they felt able to attend the project. Once they were taking part, families were assigned a key worker. Throughout the families' attendance at the project the key worker would visit the family at home every one or two weeks. The purpose of these visits differed from family to family. They might include counselling and advice on practical aspects of parenting, or they might simply help the mother to develop trust with the key worker. Key workers worked with only one family at a time. Thus the project had room for as many families as there were key workers. In the past when a member of staff had been a key worker for two families this had caused problems in the group. This was because in some respects key workers became parent figures for some mothers and thus shared key workers could lead to 'sibling' rivalry within the group.

The PP team included an occupational therapist, a community psychiatric nurse, a counsellor, a nursing assistant, a health visitor, a crèche worker, a music therapist, a social worker and a group therapist. Great emphasis was placed on teamwork in the project. Although each mother would have a particular member of staff as her key worker that person would discuss the work with the team. This enabled the staff team to support one another and also to prevent families from splitting the staff members into 'good' and 'bad' workers.

The parents and children attended the project one day a week, from 9.30am to 2pm. The project was run in six-week blocks, with a review every seventh week. Families attended for an average of six months. Some came for a shorter time and the maximum was about 12 months. The day was generally structured as follows:

9.30 – 10.00	Arrive
10.00 – 11.00	Group 1
11.00 – 11.15	Coffee
11.15 – 12.00	Group 2
12.00 – 12.45	Lunch
12.45 – 14.00	Parents' Support Group (children looked after by staff)

The two groups in the morning covered different aspects of parenting. These groups were sometimes with the whole family, or on other occasions the staff looked after the children while the parents worked together as a group. Activities with the children included art, cooking, play and music therapy. The Parents' Support Group ran every week. Topics for discussion included assertiveness, temper tantrums, anxiety management or relationships. Sometimes parents would gain much from hearing that other families were struggling and then felt less isolated in their difficulties. At other times, staff worked hard not to allow one family to dominate the entire session. Sometimes friendships were formed, but on other occasions tensions existed between families.

No family was ever forced to leave the PP. The timing of the leaving was a result of discussion between the key worker and the family. Every effort was made to ensure a good ending. This was often difficult for the family because their personal experience of endings might have been be negative. Key workers encouraged families to stay until the end of a six-week block. They could also advise on employment, training courses or other social activities that might benefit the family after leaving.

Music therapy with the PP

I took part in the project for two consecutive weeks in every 6- or 12-week block, by prior arrangement with one of the PP staff team members. I initially met with staff to discuss individual difficulties and aims for each family. During the first week a music therapy group was then run with the parents and the children, and a member of the project staff. This was videoed, so that the following week could consist of a discussion with the parents, the staff member present the previous week and myself, while viewing the previous week's session on video. I would seek to help the parents in line with the overall aims in the project. After each of the two music therapy interventions I would review the session with the member of staff taking part in the group who would then feed back to the staff team to ensure that the work had an on-going value.

The particular value of the music therapy group in the PP was similar to that of the music therapy group in the MTG . However, work in the PP was much shorter. The rationale here was that parents would have a new or slightly different experience with their baby in the music therapy group, and that by reflecting on this experience they might gain some new insight into their particular difficulty. However, this insight might need to be fostered and developed through continued discussion with the key worker on the project, which is why it was essential for me to liaise so closely with project staff on each of my visits.

For example, it was not unusual for mothers to be surprised at how proud they felt watching their baby playing the drum to the group and being encouraged by a round of applause. This new-found pleasure in their child's achievements would be fed back to the key worker who might remind the mother of this feeling when thinking of positive aspects of the relationship between the mother and the child. Other mothers would be pleasantly surprised when watching themselves playing and singing with their baby on the video recording. Until that moment they had been convinced that they never had a 'nice time' with their children. Here again a key worker might well view the video of the music therapy session at a later stage with the mother to remind her that there were times in her life when she was able to enjoy her child rather than be in constant conflict.

CLARE AND CATHY

Clare was a strong-willed 18-month-old girl who liked to be in control. Her mother, Cathy, felt she spent her entire life fighting with her daughter and found life very tiring. In the music therapy group, Clare clearly loved music and was the first to make choices. She was confident and happy to perform to the group. Although I noticed Cathy struggling to hold on to Clare when we were playing instruments on the floor, I also noticed her gleam of pride when her daughter was enjoying playing for the others. The best moment came when Clare led the group from the drum and controlled everyone's playing. When Clare stopped, we all stopped. Here Clare was in control in a positive way and she was obviously delighted. When reviewing the video, Cathy was able to see her daughter's need to control in a positive light for the first time. It was through watching and listening to Clare that I was able to determine that she liked and needed to feel in control of situations. However, I did not feel that she was always seeking confrontation or being deliberately naughty. I was, therefore, quite easily able to set up a situation where her strength and confidence were shown up in a positive light.

TOM AND ELISABETH

Elisabeth was a 16-year-old mother with a seven-month-old baby boy, Tom. She was reluctant to come to the group and showed adolescent embarrassment about playing any instruments herself. She did, however, agree to come for Tom's sake. Tom was very interested in my guitar-playing and watched me intently. When I started playing the piano, he started swaying to the music, and I noticed how Elisabeth was so focused on her son that she started swaying with him. Later on, she forgot herself again and started playing some bells with him, clearly enjoying the music making herself. I did not comment on her involvement in the music making during the next week's review, as I felt she was not yet ready to acknowledge this. But she was more positive about the session, saying she wanted to come again – because Tom enjoyed it so much. In this example, it was the child's natural ability to respond to music that drew the mother back into a forgotten playful mode. The mother could not resist listening to and feeling her baby's reactions to the music. Her own new or rediscovered ability to be playful then made it easier to play with her son and thus enhance their relationship.

Conclusion

In Chapter 4, I described short-term music therapy work with children with psychiatric difficulties and started off by explaining that it is still relatively unusual. In this chapter I have described short-term family music therapy work, which is even more uncommon. Nevertheless, the case studies show how effective this work can be. It has the advantage of being cost-effective because the music therapist can effect change through only a small amount of intervention. Sometimes the short-term aspect of the work can be frustrating because clients are discharged just when I feel I might be able to start being helpful. In most cases, however, potential for change can be demonstrated, which in itself is a rewarding experience and can provide clients with hope and the necessary confidence to seek further treatment.

Chapter 6

Music Therapy Research

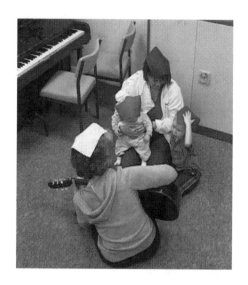

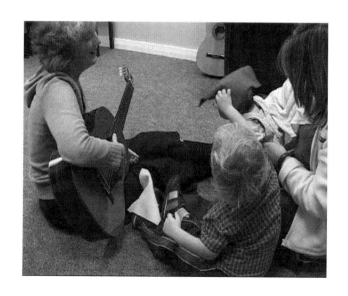

Introduction

During the past 25 years I have set up and completed four music therapy investigations. The first was with groups of adults with severe learning disabilities. That project was finished in 1986 and was awarded an MPhil by City University. The second was a smaller project with groups of mothers and pre-school children, with funding provided by Anglia Ruskin University; the writing up was completed in July 2000. The third project was with ten pre-school children on the autistic spectrum and their parents, receiving individual music therapy treatment at the Child Development Centre (Oldfield 2006). The fourth project compared Music Therapy Diagnostic Assessments (MTDAs) with Autistic Diagnostic Observation Schedules (ADOSs) at the Croft Unit for Child and Family Psychiatry. That work is described in detail in Chapter 7. The funding for these last two projects was provided by a three-year music therapy fellowship granted by the Music Therapy Charity. These two investigations formed part of my PhD, which was completed in 2003.

In this chapter I have used material from my MPhil, my PhD and several research publications (Oldfield 2000; Oldfield and Adams 1990; Oldfield *et al.* 2003).

I shall now focus briefly on the first project, dwell on how the project started, summarise the methodology and the results, and reflect on what I learnt from the investigation. This will lead me on to some thoughts about qualitative and quantitative research methodologies and about what actually constitutes research. The second investigation will then be described before reflecting on common points in all my research investigations.

Effects of music therapy on a group of adults with profound learning disabilities

How the study started

In the early 1980s I worked as a full-time music therapist at an institution for 200 people with learning difficulties. The clients varied in ages and levels of ability and I worked in a multi-disciplinary team with clinical psychologists, speech therapists, physiotherapists and occupational therapists. I treated some clients individually and some in groups, either jointly with other therapists or on my own. Although my timetable was very full, I had more referrals than I could deal with and found that I had to make difficult choices. After a few years, I noticed that I was tending to give priority to clients with very severe learning difficulties and that it seemed to be effective to treat these clients in small groups. Although I felt that this work was valuable, the responses I was getting from the clients were only small and I wanted to investigate further.

A review of the literature revealed that there was very little music therapy research in this area and none investigating the type of interactive music therapy approach used in the UK with this client group (Oldfield and Adams 1990).

The idea of setting up a research project was received with enthusiasm by my colleagues, and the clinical psychologist, Malcolm Adams, agreed to work with me. Before we started, Malcolm provided help and advice on how to fill in the Local Ethics Committee forms. Once we had received their approval we were able to proceed.

Method

We agreed that the aim of the study was to find out how effective music therapy was in achieving a set of objectives when working with a group of adults with profound learning difficulties. To answer this question we studied two groups of six clients and compared music therapy with play activities. Group A received 20 weekly music therapy sessions while group B was having play sessions; this was followed by group B receiving 20 weekly music therapy sessions while group A had play sessions.

Before starting the clinical work, staff involved in both the music therapy sessions and the play sessions agreed on three or four common objectives for each of the 12 clients involved in the research project. We decided to randomly select two clients from each of the groups for intensive study. In order to compare progress between the subjects in the two groups, we selected the experimental subjects so that they had a corresponding person in the other group with similar needs and objectives. We videotaped the experimental subjects on a weekly basis so that, by the end of the 40 experimental sessions, each of the subjects had been recorded for quarter of an hour during ten play sessions and ten music therapy sessions.

Measures

For each of the four experimental subjects we translated our clinical objectives into observable behaviours that could be timed and counted through video analysis. When the treatment was finished I analysed the 40 videotapes, viewing them in random order. I used a time-sampling method with five-second intervals to record the behaviours of both the subjects and the staff. It was necessary to record some staff behaviours because the aims for some individuals related to, for example, response to staff attention. Malcolm also analysed six of the tapes (three music and three play) at random to check that we reached an acceptable level of agreement in our analyses and that my observations were reliable.

The video-observation records provided frequency and duration measures for both client and staff behaviour in the sessions. These provided the data for the indices reflecting progress on the agreed therapy aims. Comparisons between play and music were evaluated for each individual separately using non-parametric statistics.

Results

The main hypothesis to be investigated in this study was that, for each individual, the objectives that had been specified would be achieved to a greater extent in the music therapy sessions than in the play sessions. In general the study showed that:

- all four experimental subjects showed a higher level of performance in some aspects of their behaviour in music therapy sessions

- only one experimental subject showed a higher level of performance in any aspect of her behaviour in play sessions.

These positive results were strengthened by the fact that less staff attention was needed in music therapy sessions than in play sessions to obtain higher levels of performance. However, the results were somewhat weakened by the fact that there were almost no general trends in the experimental subjects' progress in either music therapy sessions or play sessions.

Reflections on this project

Perhaps the most important aspect of this study was that it forced me to examine and question my own work in great depth. I learnt a great deal about my music therapy approach through repeated detailed video-observations. Some aspects of my clinical work were validated by this study, others I revised. I obviously learnt a considerable amount about research and gained a certain amount of confidence in my own ability to initiate and carry out further research, knowing that I would always seek advice and support from appropriate fellow clinicians.

The mid- to late 1980s was a time when many arts therapists in Great Britain seemed to be rebelling against outcome research projects such as these, and qualitative research was in fashion, so it was useful to have to think through the qualitative versus quantitative debate. Twenty years later the debate continues but with less vehemence, many clinicians agreeing that it is possible and even desirable to include both types of approach in any music therapy investigation.

Qualitative and quantitative approaches to research

According to Wheeler (1995):

> Quantitative research: ...tests theories through procedures for scientific objectivity, including careful observation of behaviour, the isolation and manipulation of variables, and hypothesis testing.
>
> Qualitative research on the other hand describes: ...a broad category of research that reflects the belief of its followers that not all that is important can be reduced to measurements, it is essential to take into account the interaction between the researcher and the participant(s) being studied, findings cannot be generalised beyond the context in which they are discovered, and values are inherent in and central to any investigation. (p.11)

Wheeler (p.12) goes on to explain that some music therapy researchers feel that all research combines elements of both qualitative and quantitative methodology and that there is no need to choose between the two models. Other music therapists feel that the two approaches reflect opposite philosophical approaches and are therefore incompatible.

Some music therapists have strongly rejected any research that means that they will have to deal with numbers. Levinge (2000) explained that when she set up her PhD research project she informed her supervisor at the outset that if anything had to be counted she would not include it in her research. On the other hand, Edwards (2002) advocated that music therapists should be familiar with, and if necessary be prepared to work within, the evidence-based medicine (EBM) research framework which draws primarily on quantitative investigations.

Bruscia (1995, p.73) writes that one option for music therapy researchers is to use a quantitative approach for those aspects of the work that lend themselves to quantification and linear thinking, and a qualitative approach for the aspects of the work that rely on interpretation and are based on interpersonal relationships. A similar point is made by Bunt and Hoskyns (2002, p.274) when they suggest that certain types of question demand certain types of research strategy. Rogers (2000, p.13) suggests that, although it may in some ways be 'more comfortable' to adhere either to a quantitative or a qualitative approach, the real world is governed by multiple contexts and there should be room for both qualitative and quantitative approaches.

Stige (2002) suggests that music therapy researchers can avoid becoming polarised either in a qualitative or a quantitative position. Towards the end of his book, he concludes that:

> the practice and study of music therapy need an inclusive and eclectic concept of truth, acknowledging the relevance of at least three perspectives: the empiricist perspective (correspondence), the hermeneutic perspective (coherence/meaning), and the pragmatic perspective (application/effect)...these arguments suggest that music therapists could make their voices heard among those who try to link science and the humanities in some way or another. (p.307)

In all my investigations I asked focused questions at the outset, which is a characteristic of a quantitative approach. Nevertheless I was always investigating my own work and was interested in how it was evolving, which is a characteristic of a qualitative approach. Although my first objective was to find out more about and improve my clinical practice (qualitative approach), I was also keen to demonstrate that music therapy was effective (quantitative approach). In spite of the fact that the four investigations I set up were quantitative in that they asked specific questions at the outset, I was not interested only in the answers to these questions. In a sense, I had a qualitative approach to these quantitative investigations because one of my main interests lay in the learning that took place through these investigations.

What constitutes research?

In a more general context the opinion as to what constitutes research also varies greatly. In the music department at Anglia Ruskin University in Cambridge, for example, the word 'research' is used very broadly and may, for instance, include studies of new ways of interpreting or analysing compositions. Conversely, many medical practitioners not only dismiss qualitative research findings, they also dismiss quantitative findings from research that does not include randomised control trials as part of its methodology. Thus, at a recent one-day conference on autism and Asperger's syndrome organised by the Royal Society of Medicine, Howlin (2003) indicated that there was no research evidence to support many interventions, including music therapy, with children on the autistic spectrum. Nevertheless, Howlin and Rutter (1989, p.248) also advise that the three research routes of biological investigation, psychological study and therapeutic innovations should be pursued simultaneously. Two general textbooks on autism (Baron-Cohen and Bolton 1993, p.70; Trevarthen *et al.* 1996, p.172) include specific sections on music therapy. It therefore appears that although the value of music therapy as a form of treatment and, as a consequence, the importance of research in music therapy is acknowledged, the current research literature is not felt to be conclusive by some professionals.

Gfeller (1995, p.56) suggests: 'In the best possible research worlds, perhaps the most compelling reason for a particular methodology in music therapy research is the philosophical framework of the researcher regarding musical response'.

Thinking about methodology and in response to Gfeller's suggestion above, my philosophical framework regarding my clients' or my own musical responses is that these responses provide the means by which I will communicate and interact with my clients. I believe that every person has the potential to interact through sounds in some way and that it is my job to find out what the client's specific ways of interacting may be. The musical responses are crucial and central to my work, but remain a vehicle rather than an aim in themselves. Thus, in my research methodology, my starting point will be the therapeutic aims or diagnostic criteria that I have for each case.

Edwards (1999a) outlines four social science approaches relevant to research in music therapy: positivism, post-positivism, constructivism and critical theory. She writes:

> What has traditionally been viewed as 'quantitative research' in the music therapy literature is arguably post-positivist because of its concern with setting and multiple testing. What has been considered 'qualitative research' is also to be positioned within the post-positivist paradigm. (p.79)

My research investigation could be described as post-positivist in that I am investigating music therapy processes as they are being practised rather than changing aspects of my work for the purposes of the research. However, my concerns with the relationship between the principal carer and the child (explored further later in this chapter) could be seen as a constructivist approach.

Other music therapy researchers have written about difficulties arising from trying to fit into an established methodological pattern. Thus Ansdell and Pavlicevic (2001, pp.97–98) suggested that researchers should avoid defending a research methodology for its own sake, but focus on the questions the research is asking and find appropriate methodologies to answer those questions.

I have developed different approaches to my research and have used a mixture of different research methods depending on whether I am reviewing literature, describing and reflecting on my work or organising and writing about the two experimental studies. I have tried to adjust my way of thinking and my methods of analysing my results to the types of question I was asking at the time. I have felt that it was important to keep in mind that I was primarily interested in evaluating my own clinical work without being constrained by established research methodologies. I have combined qualitative and quantitative approaches because this was appropriate for what I wanted to investigate.

In spite of this varied approach, I remain convinced that my research has been thorough and interesting. According to Bruscia (1995):

> Research is a systematic, self monitored inquiry which leads to a discovery or new insight which, when documented and disseminated, contributes to or modifies existing knowledge and practice. Research differs from clinical practice in the need for meta-reflection on the data, goals, roles, beneficiaries, use of knowledge, and consumers. (p.27)

I have always aimed to meet these criteria.

Investigation into music therapy with mothers and young children at a unit for child and family psychiatry

How the study started

While I was working with a four-year-old boy with Asperger's syndrome I was struck by the similarities between my interactions with him and my interactions with my ten-month-old twin baby daughters. Both interactions were mainly non-verbal and relied to some extent on intuitive and spontaneous exchanges. In both situations, the exchanges were playful and included gentle teasing, humour and laughter. Issues of control came up both with the babies and with the client (Oldfield and Cramp 1994). These striking similarities made me aware of the value of working as a music therapist with mothers and young children. I became aware of how useful musical interactions between mothers and young children could be to explore and focus on relationship difficulties. Issues of control could be addressed and mothers could rediscover how to enjoy being playful.

Once again, I was convinced this work was of value but wanted to set up a research project to focus more deeply on this area of work.

I also thought that the study would be of particular interest because it involved short-term music therapy work with mothers and young children, which is a relatively unusual area for music therapists to work in. There was only a little literature on the subject and I did not know of any outcome research.

Although I wanted to set up an experimental piece of work, I also knew that part of the value of the project would be the descriptive data. I realised that the personal experience which had led me to this piece of work was also important. In other words, the research would be qualitative as well as quantitative.

As I was now teaching at Anglia Ruskin University, I was able to get two research grants for this project. This meant we were able to employ a research assistant, the music therapist Lucy Bunce.

Method

For the experimental part of the project, we studied three different groups:

- Mothers and Toddlers Group (MTG) attending six play sessions followed by six music therapy sessions

- group of mothers and young children from the Parenting Project (PP) who took part in three one-off, videotaped music therapy sessions followed by a review the following week, involving discussing the group with the mothers while watching the previous week's session on videotape

- as a point of comparison, a group of children and their parents attending a series of six weekly music groups in a mainstream nursery.

All the clinical work that we studied remained the same as it would have been had we not being doing the research (Oldfield *et al.* 2000). In the investigation we asked the following questions:

- To what extent do the mothers and children engage in the music and play therapy?

- To what extent do the music and play sessions encourage the mothers and the children to interact with each other?

- Do the mothers and children exhibit any negative behaviours in the music and play therapy sessions?

- Are there differences between the mother's and children's behaviour in the music and play sessions?

- Are there differences between the mother's perceptions of their children's behaviours and the actual behaviours of the children?

Measures

Information on the groups was gathered in a variety of ways. All the music therapy sessions and the play sessions were videotaped and the tapes analysed using similar time sampling methods as in the study described earlier in this chapter. In addition, questionnaires were filled out by parents on a weekly basis. Audiotapes of the discussions between the parents and the therapists after each session were analysed.

Results and reflections

The experimental investigation had positive outcomes as the video analyses showed that aims and objectives initially set out for parents and children were achieved both in play sessions and in music therapy sessions. The levels of engagement by the mothers and the children were high in both settings, and the mothers and the children interacted well with one another in both play and music therapy groups.

Probably the most interesting finding was that information gathered from the video analyses, when compared with information collated from the questionnaires given to parents, showed that parents attending the Croft Unit may be influenced by how they feel about their child and might not always accurately remember what their child's behaviour was like in the session. Thus parents attending the Croft might see their child's performance as inadequate or ordinary whereas the nursery group parents would see the same behaviours in their child as exciting and interesting.

Common points in all my research investigations

Although all four projects were with very different client groups, they had a lot in common.

- In all of my research work I worked very closely with other clinicians. The clinical psychologist Malcolm Adams was my supervisor in the first project and an essential advisor in the next three. In all four projects, members of the clinical teams were very involved in the research, and in the last three a part-time music therapy research assistant was employed specifically to work on various aspects of the investigations.

- In all four projects, there was a strong emphasis on quantitative results as well as on descriptive work.

- Three out of the four projects depended on the music therapist setting clear treatment goals for her clients.

- Three out of the four projects relied heavily on video analysis.

- All four investigations arose out of music therapy practice and aimed to look at music therapy as it was practised rather than setting up clinical work especially for the investigation.

- In all four projects the researcher was investigating her own clinical work.

Reflections

Possibly the most valuable aspect of these research projects on my work as a music therapist was that I was forced to think and question the very nature of my work. As a researcher working simultaneously as a clinician, I find that my research work makes me look critically at my clinical work, viewing the music therapy processes as an outside non-music therapist might see them. On the other hand, the clinical music therapy work enables me to directly relate the research questions to clinical practice rather than taking a more distant theoretical viewpoint.

In all the projects, results were positive and encouraging but many interesting findings came unexpectedly. In the first study we compared the results from the video analyses to the descriptive method I had of writing up notes after each session. We found that the two were quite similar, indicating that my system of note-taking seemed to be effective (Oldfield 1993a). In the second study it was a comparison between results from the video analyses and parents' questionnaires that revealed interesting results. Thus it seems that it is often a side issue rather than the main issue investigated that ends up being the most interesting of all.

Carrying out research investigations can be a good way of bringing staff together. Methodology and research procedure will have to be shared and discussed. Staff will feel that their work is being valued enough to warrant investigation and will often feel renewed interest and enthusiasm for their work.

When preparing recent applications for music therapy research funding I realised that I was using systems and procedures that had been learnt from my previous four investigations. I shall now outline some of these ideas, as they may be useful to other music therapists interested in setting up research projects. These suggestions will be particularly helpful if the proposed research has points in common with the list in the previous section of this chapter (see p.120).

1. Research initially arises from clinical practice, so the researcher may find it useful to seek to answer a burning clinical issue or a question that keeps being raised.

2. The music therapy researcher should talk to other clinicians in the team about the idea of setting up a project. Do they feel it would be worth investigating, and support the project?

3. Once the ideas begin to take shape, it is useful to consult relevant literature and colleagues who may have been involved in research.

4. It is important to seek help regarding methodology from a research specialist such as a clinical psychologist, a psychiatrist, or another music therapist.

5. It is important to determine what questions need to be answered.

6. The numbers of clients or groups that need to be investigated and videotaped should be determined.

7. The length of time that the clients will be investigated should be decided.

8. Practicalities such as where the experimental work will take place, what video equipment should be used, who will videotape and who will analyse the videos should be sorted out.

9. What questionnaires, interviews or structured interviews are needed should be determined. Some existing questionnaires may be used, others may be devised specially.

10. Funding should be applied for if necessary.

11. Ethical applications will have to be filled out. This often seems a huge task but it can be helpful to plan the project clearly and write an outline of the initial research proposal. Consent forms and information sheets may need to be written.

12. Video analysis forms to analyse the video data will need to be devised, or existing forms other researchers have used may be adapted. It is essential to practise collating information from videotapes until reliable results are achieved. Random reliability checks with another observer are usually necessary.

13. Information from video analyses, questionnaires and interviews will then need to be collated and put into tables or graphs.

14. If necessary, statistical analyses should be used to look at the significance of results, if possible with specialist help.

15. Although many researchers start writing up only once the outcome investigations are completed, it is useful to keep written records of the whole research procedure from the very beginning. Qualitative descriptive data is just as important as an analysis of the figures.

Conclusion

At times research may seem a daunting prospect to working music therapists. However, it can be tremendously rewarding and will usually help and improve clinical practice.

Many of the qualities needed to be a music therapist are precisely those needed in research. Music therapists are used to having to be flexible and working as part of multidisciplinary teams, which is essential in research. However, music therapists and researchers also have to be able to work independently as well as being self-motivated and determined. Most musicians are used to boring practice routines and will be prepared for monotonous and repetitive analysis. In addition, both music therapists and researchers need to combine rigorous thinking with the ability to be creative and innovative.

Chapter 7

Research Investigation into Music Therapy Diagnostic Assessments

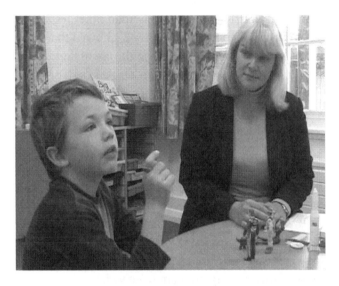

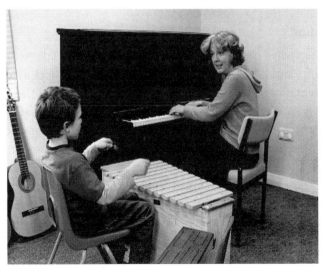

Introduction

As I have explained in Chapter 2, the Music Therapy Diagnostic Assessments (MTDAs) at the Croft Unit were developed in order to assist the clinical team with the diagnoses of the children's difficulties. At weekly management meetings at the Croft, I found that I often had opinions that were different from those of the rest of my colleagues in the team about the children on the unit, especially when assessing children with possible autistic spectrum disorder. In particular, it seemed that the MTDAs were sometimes able to find out about the children's abilities to communicate non-verbally more quickly and effectively than other tests.

The review of the literature in Chapter 2, showed that not many music therapists have written about or researched the use of music therapy to assist diagnoses. It therefore seemed logical to set up a research project in this area.

At the Croft, one of the principal tests used for children suspected of being on the autistic spectrum is the Autism Diagnostic Observation Schedule (ADOS) which is described later in this chapter under 'Measurements'. As this is a very imaginative test relying heavily on creative interactions with the tester, I thought that it would be interesting to compare the results of the MTDA to the results of the ADOS. I wanted to compare the MTDA not only to the test that was in current use at the Croft but also to a test that I felt was effective and good at capturing children's attention.

In this chapter, I first explain how this project was set up, then outline the methodology I used and go on to examine the results of the study. Finally the main findings of this investigation are reviewed.

Background

My first step when considering this investigation was to talk to the members of the Croft team. As I had worked at the unit as a music therapist since 1987, I knew the staff very well and music therapy was well-established and recognised as a valuable contribution to the work on the unit. In addition, I had already carried out the mothers and toddlers investigation (described in Chapter 6) at the Croft Unit between 1996 and 1998 and collaborated closely with members of the Croft team in this venture. The staff were, therefore, very supportive and interested in this research proposal. The consultant psychiatrist on the unit, Jo Holmes, was not only very encouraging, but agreed to fill in questionnaires after the ADOS tests and also consented to be one of my research supervisors, focusing particularly on the clinical aspects of my research investigation. It was felt that the fact that Jo Holmes was simultaneously a colleague, an assessor in the project and a research supervisor would be helpful rather than cause any difficulties. This was partly because our roles within the team were already well-defined and our two research assessments were carried out independently. Malcolm Adams, who is a clinical psychologist and currently Co-director of the Doctoral Training Programme in Clinical Psychology, University of East Anglia, agreed to act as research consultant.

Methodology

Overview of the study design

The aim of this investigation was to find out whether MTDAs were effective at highlighting important aspects of behaviour which are symptomatic of (or exclude) a diagnosis of autistic spectrum disorder.

I decided to investigate 30 children receiving ADOS and MTDA tests at the Croft Unit over a period of two years. This number was big enough to allow me to estimate the effect size of the relationship between the two assessments. In addition it was anticipated that this was the approximate number of children with suspected autistic spectrum disorder that would be admitted to the Croft in the time available for the investigation. For practical reasons, carrying out the experimental work over a period of two years meant that I would have time to analyse and write up my results within the three-year period of my research fellowship. A system of scoring MTDAs which is similar to the system used to score ADOS tests was devised. The scores for the two tests were then compared.

After each assessment the MTDA and ADOS testers were given a questionnaire regarding how effective they felt the test had been on that day for that particular child. The consultant psychiatrist, Jo Holmes, usually filled in this questionnaire for the ADOS and I completed the questionnaires about the MTDAs. Answers were collated and compared.

The children were given structured interviews after each MTDA and ADOS test by the music therapy research assistant. Results of these interviews were gathered together and compared.

Choice of the research design

This investigation was carried out at a psychiatric unit and it was therefore important that treatment and assessments proceeded as usual and that the pattern of diagnostic tests was not changed for the purposes of this investigation.

Before this investigation was started, children suspected of having autistic spectrum disorder who were admitted to the Croft would routinely receive two MTDAs and an ADOS test. The parents of the children would also be offered an Autistic Diagnostic Interview (ADI). In addition, the children and families would be assessed by the Croft team in a variety of settings such as the unit school, the Croft playground, various therapeutic groups, at meal times and (for those families who were residential) at night and in the evenings and early mornings.

I felt that I would be able to evaluate the MTDAs by comparing the results of the second of these two assessments to the results of the ADOS. I used the second of the two MTDAs because during the first MTDA the emphasis was often on familiarising the child with the musical instruments and the concept of free improvisation, whereas in the second MTDA I could focus more clearly on the diagnostic assessment. I did not consider using an average score of the two MTDA sessions because each of the MTDAs served a different function. The MTDA and the ADOS were similar enough to be compared. Nevertheless, I was aware that the final diagnosis and report that was written on each child was based not only on MTDA and ADOS results but also on the findings of the team as a whole. This is why I have also examined ADI results as well as the diagnoses written in the children's discharge reports.

I was also interested in finding out how the people doing the tests felt about the effectiveness of the assessments. I therefore devised a question-naire that was the same for both the MTDA tester and the ADOS tester. The people who administer tests usually have clear ideas about which parts of the tests are particularly useful and which questions provide interesting answers. By answering questions straight after each test, I thought I would gather interesting information, which might well give me ideas as to how to improve my MTDAs for future use.

In addition, I wanted to know what the children felt about the tests and devised a semi-structured interview for the research assistant to use with the children after the MTDA and ADOS tests. I wondered whether children found music therapy assessments unusual or intimidating and whether they enjoyed the playful nature of the ADOS tests.

My results were subjected to statistical analysis. I used the SPSS computer software to help me with my calculations and the Microsoft Excel program to draw charts and diagrams.

The children

As soon as I received ethical approval in October 2000, I started approaching the families of children admitted to the Croft who were suspected of being on the autistic spectrum, to ask whether they would consent to taking part in this research project. The Croft team told me when a new child with possible autistic spectrum disorder was admitted and gave me some basic information about the family. I then approached the child's parent or carer while they were on the unit, explained about the project, gave them the information sheet and asked them to sign the consent form. If the parent wanted time to think about giving consent I suggested that she or he could return the consent form on the following day. Sometimes, I saw the parent and the child at the same time and I showed the child the special information sheet for children and asked the child to sign the children's consent form. At other times, particularly when the child had obvious difficulties with reading and writing, I asked the parent to go over the information sheet for the child at another time and suggested that the child might like to draw a cross or a picture on the consent form. On a few occasions, when I was not available at the right time, another member of the Croft team went through the information sheets and consent forms with the families.

Although more than two out of three of the children on this project were diagnosed as being either on the autistic spectrum or borderline autistic spectrum, all these children were verbal and most of them attended mainstream school and were not severely learning disabled. It is possible that clear diagnoses had not been made previously because of the relatively high abilities of these children.

Figure 7.1 Ratio of girls to boys illustrates that the majority of the 30 children seen during this research project were male with only five girls compared to 25 boys. The children varied in age from four to twelve.

Figure 7.2 shows that although the children were fairly well distributed in terms of their ages, there were slightly more between the ages of seven to nine and ten to twelve than in the younger bracket between four and six.

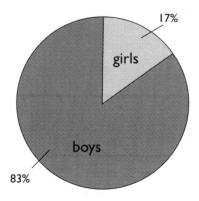

Figure 7.1 Ratio of girls to boys

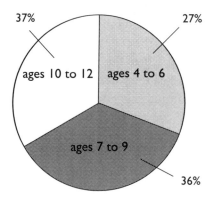

Figure 7.2 Age distribution of the children

Measurements

ADOS

Lord *et al.* (1989) mention several different observational scales for the diagnosis of autism such as the Behaviour Observations Scale for Autism (BOS) (Freeman *et al.* 1984) and the Autism Observation Scale (Siegel *et al.* 1986). However, they point out that these scales 'are less effective in identifying higher functioning autistic children and adolescents than autistic children who are severely handicapped' (Lord *et al.* 1989, p.187).

The ADOS was originally developed to discriminate autistic children aged from six years onwards with mild or no mental handicap from children with matched intelligence quotients (IQs) who were not autistic (Lord *et al.* 1989). Over the years the test has evolved slightly and the current version used in this investigation is a little different from the one originally described by Lord and co-worker.

There were two aspects of the ADOS which made it different from other diagnostic tests and which were also the reason that it was a good test to use as a comparison for my new MTDA. These were (a) that the ADOS was an *interactive* schedule, and (b) that it allowed the rating of the *quality* of social behaviour and not just its absence or its occurrence in limited quantities. The ADOS presents the child with a range of different social situations to which to react. In each situation, the ADOS examiner will interact with the child to elicit certain target responses. As a result, the ADOS can be administered only by people who have experience of interacting with children with autistic spectrum disorder, and who are specially trained to use this test (Lord *et al.* 1989).

The ADOS test varies slightly depending on how old and how verbal the child is. Different levels or modules of the test are used depending on ability levels. In 1995 Dilavore and co-workers adapted the ADOS for pre-linguistic children and called it the Pre-linguistic Autism Diagnostic Observation Schedule (PL-ADOS) (Dilavore *et al.* 1995). General ratings are made on a three-point scale:

0 = within normal limits

1 = infrequent or possible abnormality

2 = definite abnormality.

The ratings are made in four areas:

A: communication/language

B: reciprocal social interaction

C: imagination/creativity

D: stereotyped/restricted behaviours.

Sections A and B are considered by the authors of the test to be the most successful in predicting diagnosis. Nevertheless, sections C and D are also looked at carefully because they are clinically relevant.

All the children who had the ADOS test in this research investigation were verbal, so module 3 for children who are verbally fluent was used.

There were 12 activities in the ADOS (13 activities if you include the break). Although the break was not an activity as such, the child was assessed during this free period even though the tester appeared to be writing notes and not observing the child. However, the scoring system does not relate directly to these activities but rather to specific difficulties that might become apparent through these activities. The 12 activities were:

- construction task
- make-believe play
- joint interactive play
- demonstration task
- description of picture
- conversation/non-routine event
- cartoons
- story from a book
- emotions
- social difficulties/divergence
- friends, relationships, loneliness
- creating a story.

More details on the ADOS scoring procedure are included in Lord *et al.* 1989. The 11 points that are scored on the ADOS scoring sheet are listed under two categories: (1) communication and (2) qualitative impairments in reciprocal social interaction. For both these categories an 'autism' cut-off point and an 'autistic spectrum' cut-off point were indicated.

MTDS

The MTDA has been described in detail in Chapter 2. For this research investigation I had to devise a way of scoring these assessments that could be compared to the scoring system used in the ADOS.

Like the ADOS test, the MTDA includes various activities; but although some activities are included in every assessment the choice of activities is adapted to each child and varies slightly from assessment to assessment. Occasionally an activity might be repeated.

For most children, eight or nine of the activities listed on pages 37–38 are included in the MTDA. Activities marked with a star are almost always included in the sessions; three or four of the other activities are chosen depending on each child's preferences, strengths and weaknesses.

In order to decide how to score these assessments, I tried to formulate questions that I felt I was able to answer through these activities rather than evaluate each activity individually. The experience of having tried out these MTDAs over a number of years at the Croft was invaluable at this stage. Having discussed many children who had been through MTDAs with the team, I already had some clear ideas about what types of information I felt my assessments were good or quick at gaining about the children. I was also particularly interested in pinpointing those areas where I felt I often disagreed with the other assessments that had been carried out on the unit.

After several attempts and trials and much debate with other members of the Croft team I came up with a scoring system that I used for the 30 children involved in this research investigation (Appendix 7). The full MTDA gathers information on other areas of difficulty the children may be experiencing which may not be symptomatic of autistic spectrum disorder. Although I will be studying only questions (a) to (l) in this investigation, I had to answer all the questions for all the children as my research work overlapped with my clinical work at the Croft. As a clinician I needed to reflect on the children's general strengths and weaknesses in order to feed back more clearly to the team in management meetings at the end of the week.

The score cut-off points were chosen to be similar to the cut-off points in the ADOS test. The cut-off point for autism was set at 6, and the cut-off point for autistic spectrum disorder which would include Asperger's syndrome and Pervasive Developmental Disorder of a non-specific type (PDD-NOS), was set at 10. It must be remembered that this scoring system was developed especially for this investigation and has not been tested or tried out in great depth. I expect that in the future the scoring system will be modified and improved as more music therapists try to use it. (See Appendix 7, first part of the MTDA, relevant to autism.)

Comparison between MTDA and ADOS tests

There were some obvious similarities and differences between the MTDA and the ADOS tests and scoring systems.

Both tests lasted 30–45 minutes and focused on the interactions between the tester and the child. The ADOS test focused on interactions through play and through verbal interactions. The MTDA focused on interactions through music making. The module-3 ADOS test we were using in this investigation probably included more verbal interactions than the MTDA.

Although the ADOS test was interactive and playful, some parts of the assessment could be seen by the child as being quite like a traditional test where the child is presented with a construction task or a puzzle to complete. In reality, the tester was not concerned with whether or not the task was completed but more with how the child approached the task and if he or she spontaneously sought help from the adult. Similarly, some children expected the music therapist to teach them a tune or how to play an instrument. Again the tester was more interested in the process of learning rather than the acquisition of a skill.

In both the ADOS and the MTDA the child may have preconceived ideas about what will happen in the assessments. In the ADOS, which at the Croft is usually administered by a medical doctor, the child may assume that he or she will be medically examined or asked questions about his or her health. In the MTDA the child may expect to be taught a musical instrument or asked to sing.

There were some very obvious overlaps between the ADOS and the MTDA. For example, in both tests the children were asked to make up a story.

The ADOS test was a one-off test whereas the MTDA was done over two half-hour sessions usually held on a weekly basis. Nevertheless it was decided that for the purposes of this investigation only the second MTDA would be used and scored. The first MTDA was felt to fulfil the function of familiarising the child with the musical equipment and the somewhat unfamiliar process of improvising freely with the tester. However, the fact that the child would have already met the music therapist and would have had an MTDA did not bias the results in favour of music therapy for the purpose of the investigation. This was because the child would also usually have met and become familiar with the person carrying out the ADOS at outpatient and pre-admission appointments. In both the ADOS and MTDA, the person carrying out the test was a member of the Croft team but not one of the main nursing staff. So the child would have seen and met the adult who carried out the test but would not have known the person very well.

The ADOS always included the same 13 activities although occasionally an activity might be left out, sometimes due to time constraints and sometimes because a child was particularly unco-operative. The MTDA usually included around nine or ten activities but, although five core activities were almost always included, the others varied from child to child.

In the ADOS, all the activities were suggested by the tester, and the activities were presented in a set sequence. However, there could be flexibility within each of the activities and the tester may have been able to give the child the impression that he or she was making a choice. In the MTDA, the child and the tester took it in turns to choose activities and the *way* the child made these choices was a central part of the test.

Both the ADOS tests and the MTDAs were videotaped. The room where the ADOS was held had a camera on the wall which was operated from another room, whereas the MTDAs were videotaped by the research assistant, who was in a corner of the room with the child and the tester.

The scoring systems for the ADOS and MTDAs also had some points in common. In both scoring systems most of the questions related to ways in which the child was communicating and interacting with the adult. In the MTDA scoring system, however, questions (d), (h) and (e) which related to unusual use of objects or stereotyped forms of playing the instruments were included in the main part of the test. In the ADOS, on the other hand, the questions relating to these areas were outside the core part of the scoring system. Nevertheless, the first question in the ADOS system included stereotypes and idiosyncratic use of words and phrases, and as the MTDA focused mainly on musical rather than verbal forms of communication it seemed logical to include this aspect in the main body of the MTDA scoring system.

Table 7.1 shows how questions from the MTDA scoring system (second column) overlap or correspond in some way with questions from the ADOS scoring system (first column). Sometimes the questions asked do not match up exactly but might be looking at similar types of difficulties.

The letters and numbers that appear at the beginning of the ADOS categories refer to the code used for that category in the ADOS scoring sheet.

In this table I have tried to look at similarities in the individual categories scored in the ADOS and the MTDA assessments. Some categories such as (2) (A7) – reporting of events – in the ADOS do not have an equivalent area in the MTDA. When categories do not match up specifically to one another I have sometimes grouped questions together. On several occasions I have matched the same MTDA question to different ADOS categories because the MTDA question seemed to cover both the ADOS areas. For example, (c) in the MTDA is matched both to (3) as well as (12) in the ADOS.

Table 7.1   Overlaps and similarities between the categories in the ADOS and MTDA scoring systems

ADOS scoring categories	MTDA scoring categories
1. (A4) Stereotyped/idiosyncratic use of words or phrases	(f) Unusual or repetitive quality of tone of voice/intonation (h) Obsessive/repetitive types of playing or patterns in story
2. (A7) Reporting of events	–
3. (A8) Conversation	(c) Lack of spontaneous musical or verbal suggestions with communicative intent; inability to be creative
4. (A9) Descriptive; conventional; instrumental gestures	(b) Lack of facial or physical engagement in playing process; unusual eye-contact
5. (B1) Unusual eye-contact	–
6. (B2) Facial expressions directed to others	–
7. (B6) Insight	–
8. (B7) Quality of social overtures	(k) Child wants session to be on his/her terms
9. (B8) Quality of social response	(l) No communicative response to therapist's singing (j) Difficulties having playful or humorous exchanges with adult (g) Difficulties making up shared story
10. (B9) Amount of reciprocal social communication	(i) Child is unable to have more than one immediate copying response; exchanges do not develop into a dialogue
11. (B10) Overall quality of rapport	(a) Child's playing independent of therapist's playing

ADOS scoring categories	MTDA scoring categories
12. (C1) Imagination; creativity	(c) Lack of spontaneous musical or verbal suggestions with communicative intent; inability to be creative
13. (D1) Unusual sensory interest in play material/person	(d) Unusual interest in structure or shapes of instruments; lining up beaters, twiddling shakers
14. (D2) Hand and finger and other complex mannerisms	(e) Child is self-absorbed and difficult to distract from certain instruments
15. (D4) Excessive interest in highly specific topics or objects	(h) Child develops obsessive/repetitive styles of playing or telling stories
16. (D5) Compulsions and rituals	

The MTDA (b) was not matched up with the ADOS (6) in spite of the fact that both categories looked at unusual eye-contact, because the ADOS category looks specifically at how the child links eye-contact with speech. However, ADOS (4) and MTDA (b) both refer to non-verbal physical communication and are therefore paired up in this table.

Similarly ADOS (6) relates specifically to facial expressions directed towards other people rather than general use of facial expression to show intent or involvement which is more the focus of MTDA (b).

Only the first 11 questions in the ADOS form part of the scores that determine the autism and autistic spectrum cut-off scores. However, questions 12 to 16 are always scored and will form part of the descriptive data when reporting back about the test.

I shall be referring back to this table in the results section of this chapter.

Testers' questionnaires

In addition to gathering information about the children's strengths and weaknesses from the MTDA and ADOS scoring sheets, I thought it would be useful for the people administering the tests to fill in a questionnaire after the session. In this questionnaire, the people administering the tests (myself and usually the consultant psychiatrist, Jo Holmes) answered questions about how useful they felt each individual activity within the test had been. I devised a form where each of the activities in the test could be listed and evaluated in the following way: 'a' (4) for very effective; 'b' (3) for effective; 'c' (2) for not very informative, or 'd' (1) for useless.

On the second page of the form there were three more general questions which were:

- Did the person carrying out the test feel that they administered the test well?

- What were the limitations of the test?

- Particular immediate impressions of child: what stood out?

Finally there was a question for staff members who might have been observing the test. This asked whether the child behaved in an expected or unexpected way during the session. A blank tester's questionnaire is included as Appendix 8.

Although an attempt was made to fill in the forms straight after the sessions, this was not always possible. Nevertheless, we were able to use the test results, children's notes and video recordings of the sessions to help us remember our impressions when our memories needed to be refreshed.

Children's structured interviews

After each MTDA and ADOS, the research assistant asked each of the children some questions about the session they had just had. For a few children, when the research assistant was not available, another member of staff from the Croft did the interviews after she had explained the procedure to them.

In spite of our efforts, not all the children were interviewed after the MTDA and ADOS experimental sessions. This was because some children were reluctant to be interviewed and also because it was not always possible to find a member of staff who was available to interview the children.

I felt that it was important for the research assistant rather than the music therapist (myself) to carry out these interviews as the child was more likely to give true answers to a neutral person rather than to the person who had just run a music therapy diagnostic assessment with them.

The research assistant conducted interviews after each of the two MTDA sessions and after the ADOS test. As I am mainly using the data from the second MTDA session for this research project, I will include only the data from the second MTDA children's interviews here. Had I known at the beginning of the investigation that I would be analysing only the second MTDA sessions, I probably would not have arranged for the research assistant to conduct an interview after the first MTDA session. Having the two interviews after the MTDA sessions had the advantage of keeping the two sessions similar in structure for the children. However, it had the slight disadvantage that some questions that were included in the post-ADOS test were left out in the interview following the second MTDA sessions, because the child answered the same questions the previous week after the first MTDA session. An example of such a question might have been 'Have you done these types of activity before, at school or at home?' Nevertheless, this was not a major difficulty as most of the questions related directly to the session that had just occurred.

I devised a sheet with questions for these interviews which is included as Appendix 9. It is important to note, however, that these sheets were only used as guidelines. Often, the research assistant had to work hard to maintain the children's interest and questions would sometimes be left out if it was felt they were not appropriate for a particular child.

Results of the study

Table 7.2 shows the adjusted MTDA scores (see Appendix 7 for details of the scoring system), the ADOS scores and the Croft diagnosis for each child. The MTDA scores were adjusted because the MTDA had 12 questions and the main ADOS had 11 questions. To compare the two sets of figures, MTDA scores were divided by 12 and multiplied by 11. Figures were rounded up to the nearest half point.

The last column translates the Croft diagnoses into numerical form. In consultation with the psychiatrist, Jo Holmes, it was decided that the children with PDD-NOS diagnoses as well as some of the children with described diagnoses rather than clear labels would be grouped together as borderline children. I discussed each of the possible borderline children with Jo Holmes before deciding whether to fit them into the borderline (1) category or the ASD (2) category.

Before comparing the MTDAs, the ADOS tests and the Croft diagnoses, I looked at whether the MTDA and the ADOS tests were reliably differentiating between the three different diagnoses reached by the Croft on discharge.

Significance tests on the diagnoses reached from ADOS and MTDA scores
The data from Table 7.2 was entered into spreadsheets in the SPSS computer program and subjected to tests. I used mostly non-parametric statistical tests

Table 7.2   Music therapist's MTDA adjusted scores, main ADOS scores and diagnosis

Child	MTDA adjusted cut-off: Aut: 9 ASD: 5.5	ADOS cut-off: Aut:10 ASD:7	Croft diagnosis on discharge, or description from form	Diagnosis (numerical) 0 = no ASD 1 = Borderline 2 = ASD
C1	3.5	6	Atypical autism	1
C2	5.5	6	No ASD	0
C3	3.5	12	ASD	2
C4	4.5	9	Asperger's syndrome	2
C5	6	4	Difficulties overlap with ASD at milder end	1
C6	1	3	No ASD	0
C7	5	4	'Development consistent with ASD – atypical in his highly developed imagination'	1
C8a	3	1	No ASD	0
C9s	5.5	8	PDD-NOS	1
C10s	3.5	9	PDD-NOS	1
C11s	4	9	PDD-NOS	1
C12	6.5	*	'No ADOS, ADI indicated PDD'	2
C13	7.5	2	No PDD	0
C14	6	7	Asperger's syndrome	2
C15a	2.5	1	No ASD	0
C16	6.5	14	PDD	2
C17	7	12	Asperger's syndrome	2

Child	MTDA adjusted cut-off: Aut: 9 ASD: 5.5	ADOS cut-off: Aut:10 ASD:7	Croft diagnosis on discharge, or description from form	Diagnosis (numerical) 0 = no ASD 1 = Borderline 2 = ASD
C18	12	8	'High functionning ASD'	1
C19	2.5	11	No ASD	0
C20a	3.5	4	'Closest category would probably be PDD-NOS'	1
C21	5	6	PDD-NOS	1
C22	3	2	PDD-NOS	1
C23	4.5	4	No ASD	0
C24	5	3	PDD-NOS	1
C25	6	8	PDD-NOS	1
C26	7	10	'High functioning autism with atypical presentation'	2
C27	5.5	12	PDD-NOS	1
C28	9	14	Childhood autism	2
C29	2.5	7	PDD-NOS	1
C30a	6	7	Borderline ASD	1

* It was not possible to score this test for child C12.

because the ADOS and MTDA scores were not evenly distributed. Table 7.3 shows the mean and the standard deviations of the scores. It is encouraging to find that the mean for the three diagnostic categories rises progressively with the severity of the diagnoses for both the MTDA and the ADOS tests.

I then applied the Kruskal–Wallis test to these results. Siegel (1956) gives advice to researchers regarding which are the most appropriate signifi-cance tests to use. This test was used to determine whether the scores reached were differentiating between the three diagnostic categories in numerically

Table 7.3   **SPSS descriptive statistics on the MTDA and ADOS figures relating to the Croft diagnoses**

	Croft diagnosis		
	No ASD (0)	Borderline (1)	ASD (2)
MTDA			
Numbers	7	15	8
Mean	3.79	5.07	6.25
Standard deviation	2.20	2.24	1.67
ADOS			
Numbers	7	15	7
Mean	4.00	6.47	11.14
Standard deviation	3.56	2.70	2.61

significant ways. The aim of this test was to eliminate the possibility that the results occurred by chance.

The results of the test showed that for both the ADOS and the MTDA the scores relating to the three diagnoses are significantly different at the level $p < 0.05$ (i.e. 5%). With probability tests it is generally accepted that when $p < 0.05$ the results are significant.

This was not surprising for the ADOS, which is an established assessment tool, but very encouraging for the MTDA which we were investigating here. This result showed that the MTDA was clearly differentiating between the three diagnostic categories in a way that corresponded to the Croft diagnosis given to children on discharge.

Comments on the three diagnoses

Figure 7.3 shows the overall Croft diagnoses for the 30 children investigated: 50 per cent of the children had borderline diagnoses, 23 per cent were not on the autistic spectrum, and 27 per cent had a diagnosis of autistic spectrum disorder.

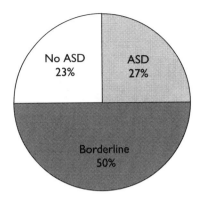

Figure 7.3 Croft diagnosis

Table 7.4   Summary of agreements and disagreements between tests

	MTDA and ADOS	MTDA and Croft	ADOS and Croft	MTDA, ADOS and Croft	MTDA or ADOS and Croft
Number where tests agree	21 (72%)	19 (63%)	19 (65%)	16 (55%)	24 (83%)
Number where tests disagree	8 (28%)	11 (37%)	10 (35%)	13 (45%)	5 (17%)

Table 7.4 summarises the agreements and disagreements between the different tests. The total numbers of children in each column sometimes add up to 29; one of the children refused to co-operate in any way in the ADOS test and could therefore not be scored for that.

The first column in this table shows that the MTDA and ADOS diagnoses agreed for 21 out of 29 children. This is further illustrated in Figure 7.4.

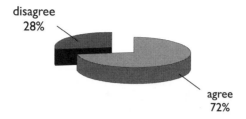

Figure 7.4 MTDA and ADOS agreements and disagreements

Despite this, Table 7.4 also indicates that neither the ADOS nor the MTDA scores always matched up with the Croft diagnosis given to the child on discharge. Nineteen out of 29 ADOS scores matched up with the diagnoses and 19 out of 30 MTDA scores matched up with the diagnoses. This observation is illustrated in Figure 7.5.

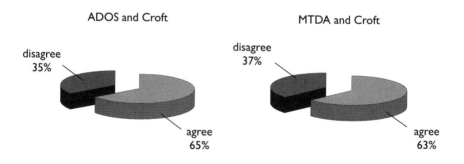

Figure 7.5 Analysis of agreements and disagreements

It is interesting to note from these charts that the percentage of agreement reached by the MTDA was very similar to that reached by the ADOS. This shows that the Croft team took the results of the relatively new MTDAs as seriously as those of the more established ADOS test.

It is also interesting to note from Table 7.4 that the agreement between the MTDA and ADOS was higher than the agreements between the Croft diagnoses and either of these two tests. Perhaps this is an indication that these tests are quite similar to one another, or at least more similar to one another than to other forms of assessment performed at the Croft.

Only 16 out of 29 children had MTDA and ADOS scores that *both* matched up with the diagnoses they were given (see Table 7.4). In one way this is not surprising as the Croft global diagnosis is very different from the individual MTDA and ADOS tests and consists of a combination of assessments. These assessments include the MTDA and the ADOS tests as well as interviews with the parents of the children and observations of the children by nursing staff and teachers in a wide variety of settings. On the other hand, it might have been expected that the consultant psychiatrist who makes the final decision about the Croft diagnosis would be more influenced by the ADOS test, which she usually administered herself. What these findings show is that the MTDA and the ADOS are only a part of the whole picture at the Croft and that many other factors and informal evaluations will influence the final diagnoses given.

It was also interesting to note that the children we most often disagreed about tended to be those with borderline diagnoses. The Croft diagnosis, the ADOS and the MTDA tended to coincide for the autistic and non-autistic diagnoses. This confirms that children who are borderline are the most difficult to diagnose.

The final column of Table 7.4 is illustrated in Figure 7.6. This shows that there were only 17 per cent of children for whom the Croft diagnosis did not agree with either the MTDA or the ADOS results. Clearly the Croft works as a team, takes note of each different assessment but considers each child carefully before deciding which pieces of information should be used for the diagnosis.

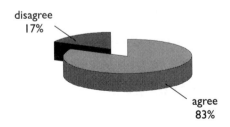

Figure 7.6 Agreement and disagreement between MTDA or ADOS with the Croft diagnosis

Analysis of MTDA and ADOS scores

I shall now look more closely at the actual scores from the MTDA and ADOS tests and subject some of these to statistical analysis. The descriptive statistical SPSS data is included in Table 7.5, which is derived from Table 7.1 earlier in this chapter. This shows that the mean score for the ADOS (7.00) is higher than the mean score for the MTDA (5.08).

Table 7.5   Summary of general statistics on the MTDA and ADOS scores

	Number of children	Mean score	Standard deviation
MTDA	30	5.08	2.21
ADOS	29	7.00	3.81

I next used the Wilcox on signed ranks test to look at whether there was a significant difference between the MTDA and ADOS scores. This test showed that the chances of these results occuring by chance were very small ($p = 0.012$). As p is smaller than 0.05, the difference between the ADOS and the MTDA results is statistically significant. As the mean showed, the ADOS scores are higher than the MTDA results. In other words, the ADOS is scoring more autistic behaviours than the MTDA.

This result, combined with the comments on the different diagnoses in the previous sub-section, confirms that the MTDA is providing different information from the ADOS for the Croft diagnostic team. This information could confirm the hypothesis that the MTDA is picking up on the children's non-verbal types of communication and is therefore less likely to judge that the child's behaviour is autistic. In order to find out where the differences between the two tests lie, I shall now compare groups of questions from each of the two assessments.

Analysis of sub-sections of MTDA and ADOS

Table 7.1 (earlier in this chapter) shows the overlaps and similarities between categories in the ADOS and MTDA scoring systems. Nine groups of questions from the ADOS and the MTDA were similar enough to be compared, so I subjected the scores from these to statistical analysis (Table 7.6).

Table 7.6   Nine similar scoring categories in MTDA and ADOS tests (from Table 7.1)

ADOS scoring categories	MTDA scoring categories
1. (A4) Stereotyped/idiosyncratic use of words or phrases	(f) Unusual or repetitive quality of tone of voice/intonation (h) Obsessive/repetitive types of playing or patterns in story
3. (A8) Conversation	(c) Lack of spontaneous musical or verbal suggestions with communicative intent; inability to be creative
4. (A9) Descriptive; conventional; instrumental gestures	(b) Lack of facial or physical engagement in playing process; unusual eye-contact
8. (B7) Quality of social overtures	(k) Child wants session to be on his or her terms
9. (B8) Quality of social response	(l) No communicative response to therapist's singing (j) Difficulties having playful or humorous exchanges with adult (g) Difficulties making up shared story
10. (B9) Amount of reciprocal social communication	(i) Child is unable to have more than one immediate copying response; exchanges do not develop into a dialogue
11. (B10) Overall quality of rapport	(a) Child's playing independent of therapist's playing
12. (C1) Imagination; creativity	(c) Lack of spontaneous musical or verbal suggestions with communicative intent; inability to be creative

ADOS scoring categories	MTDA scoring categories
13. (D1) Unusual sensory interest in play material/person	d) Unusual interest in structure or shapes of instruments; lining up beaters, twiddling shakers
14. (D2) Hand and finger and other complex mannerisms	(e) Child is self-absorbed and difficult to distract from certain instruments
15. (D4) Excessive interest in highly specific topics or objects	(h) Child develops obsessive/repetitive styles of playing or telling stories
16. (D5) Compulsions and rituals	

I applied the Wilcox signed ranks test to each of the nine lines in this table. Seven of the pairs of categories showed no significant differences in their ADOS and MTDA scores. Two pairs of categories showed significant differences in the ADOS and MTDA scores. These were:

- ADOS category 8 corresponding to MTDA category (k), looking at social overtures by the children.

- ADOS categories 13, 14, 15 and 16 corresponding to MTDA categories (d), (e) and (h), looking at ritualistic/obsessive behaviour.

I also applied descriptive statistical tests to these two pairs of categories. Results showed that the mean score for the ADOS questions in the first pair was higher than the MTDA score, whereas it was lower for the second pair. More detailed results and tables are included in my PhD thesis (Oldfield 2004).

In some ways this confirms the original idea that the MTDA is seeing more non-ASD communicative behaviours in children than is the ADOS. However, as children may be more engaged and communicative in the MTDA sessions they also might let down their defences more and display more ritualistic and obsessive behaviours, as is suggested by the data from the second of the two significantly different categories. It might also be that the music making is more stimulating and exciting than play situations and that the children show more obsessive behaviours as they become more stimulated.

MTDA and ADOS testers' questionnaires
RESULTS COLLATED FROM THE MTDA TESTERS' QUESTIONNAIRES

Although the number of activities I used in the MTDA sessions varied from four to eleven, I usually included about eight or nine activities. Some activities such as the 'hello activity', 'the act of choosing', 'large percussion and piano', 'instrumental dialogues' and 'goodbye activity' were used almost every week, whereas other activities were used only occasionally. Two activities, 'improvised story' and 'teaching a tune', were consistently felt to be very useful to the diagnostic process.

RESULTS COLLATED FROM THE ADOS TESTERS' QUESTIONNAIRES

The ADOS (schedule three was used here as the children were verbal) varied less than the MTDAs and were almost always the same every week. Sometimes, when children were very resistant to being tested or when there were time pressures, a few of the activities were left out, or the order in which the activities were presented was slightly changed.

COMMENTS ON AND COMPARISON OF TESTERS' QUESTIONNAIRE RESULTS

A blank questionnaire is included in Appendix 8. Results are summarised here; more detailed results and tables are included in my PhD thesis (Oldfield 2004).

Question 1: Was the test an effective tool?

Testers of MTDA scores and ADOS scores thought that most of the activities they used were useful for diagnostic purposes.

I subjected the mean of the scores for each of the children to statistical analysis. The results show that my scores were significantly higher than those on the ADOS test. This indicates that I felt my test was slightly more effective than the ADOS tester thought her test was. In some ways this is understandable because I was enthusiastic about my new MTDA assessment procedure. On the other hand, I knew the psychiatrist carrying out the ADOS was also convinced by the value of the ADOS test and had noticed excitement and interest on her part when I observed her carrying out these tests before this investigation began.

The ADOS included more activities in each test than did the MTDA. This is interesting as I was slightly concerned that I was trying to include too many things in my test rather than spending time encouraging a child to spend more time on individual activities in a more traditional music therapy way. It was reassuring to find that the ADOS included even more activities than the MTDA.

Question 2: Did the person carrying out the test feel they administered the test well? Answer yes or no and then comment

The prevalence of 'yes' in the questionnaires shows that both the ADOS and the MTDA testers generally felt that they administered the test well. However, the ADOS tester did answer 'no' on six occasions (out of a total of 28 answers) whereas the MTDA tester (myself) answered 'not sure' on only two occasions (out of a total of 30 answers).

The comments in this section vary greatly. It is not surprising that many of the comments made were questioning the ways in which the testers were carrying out the test as comments would probably not have been added here if the tester felt that the test had been totally straightforward to carry out. This probably explains why comments were made only about some of the children.

Table 7.7 shows an attempt to categorise the comments made as 'negative' (N), 'bland' (B) or 'positive' (P). There appear to have been more negative comments made about the ADOS test than about the MTDA test. From this table it appears that the MTDA tester (myself) had a more positive outlook regarding her test than did the ADOS tester. However, it must be remembered that although the consultant psychiatrist (Jo Holmes) did most of the ADOS tests, a number of the ADOS tests were done by senior registrars in training. It is, therefore, understandable that these senior registrars might have been less confident about administering the test than I was about administering the MTDA.

Question 3: What were the limitations of the test?

ADOS testers commented that the test was often difficult to administer because children refused to take part and were very oppositional. This difficulty was only mentioned once by the MTDA tester. ADOS testers also mentioned that some children had trouble focusing for the entire test. Conversely, other children needed more time than the test allowed to answer all the questions fully. Another subject that came up several times in the ADOS test was specific difficulties that children experienced with the verbal parts.

In some ways it is understandable that most of these difficulties were not mentioned in relationship to the MTDA. The MTDA is less clearly structured than the ADOS and can be much more child-led than the ADOS. Thus, children who like to feel they are in control would struggle less and find it easier to focus in a setting where they had more choice and leadership. In

Table 7.7   Nature of the comments made in answer to the
question: 'Did the person carrying out the test feel they
administered the test well?'

ADOS		MTDA	
Child	Type of comment	Child	Type of comment
C1	N	C1	P
C2	N	C2	P
C3	N	C3	P
C5	N	C7	N
C12	N	C9s	P
C13	N	C16	N
C15	P	C18	N
C16	N	C22	N
C21	B	C23	B
C22	N		
C23	N		
C28	N		

addition, there are more opportunities to interact and communicate non-verbally for those children who struggle with language.

A difficulty that was mentioned in the MTDAs but not in the ADOS tests was the fact that some children felt embarrassed and self-conscious. This is easily explained as some children would find it difficult not to feel they were performing when playing musical instruments.

Question 4: Particular immediate impressions of child?

This question was answered for almost all the children. I will attempt to draw out important themes by listing the children's strengths and difficulties that were often mentioned (Tables 7.8 and 7.9).

**Table 7.8   Children's strengths and difficulties mentioned
by the ADOS testers**

Strengths	Difficulties
Good conversation	Difficulties with verbal language
Chatty	Lack of social language
Sociable	Difficulties with social awareness
Good sense of humour	Lack of social understanding
Creative/imaginative	Lack of imagination
Good insight	Lack of insight
Socially approaching	Anxious/inhibited
Very articulate	Learning difficulties; socially immature
Lots of facial expressions	Controlling/rigid/stuck
Good eye-contact	Hyperactive; lack of concentration
Co-operative	Oppositional/unco-operative

Clearly there are a lot of similarities in the themes mentioned by the ADOS and the MTDA testers. However, it appears that in the ADOS there is a greater emphasis on spoken language and the MTDA tester focuses more specifically on various aspects of non-verbal communication. The MTDA tester also focuses more on the spontaneity (or lack of spontaneity) in the children, whereas the ADOS testers pick up on the children's abilities (or lack of abilities) in social understanding.

Question 5: Reaction of research assistant regarding whether child behaved in an expected or unexpected way during the session (only relevant to MTDAs)

As the research assistant was present during most of the MTDAs, videotaping the sessions, and as she saw all the children at the Croft for weekly group music therapy sessions, she was able to answer this question. As well as giving us additional information about the MTDAs this also gave us some insight into the different ways in which children might behave in group and individual music therapy sessions. Results showed that out of the 20 children

Table 7.9   Children's strengths and difficulties mentioned by the MTDA tester

Strengths	Difficulties
Communicative	Not communicative; no dialogues
Able to copy and initiate	Unable to sustain communication
Spontaneous; free in playing	No spontaneity/stuck
Interactive	Speech difficulties
Warm/affectionate	Emotional difficulties/anxious
Humorous/playful; sense of fun	Lack of confidence; self-conscious
Creative/imaginative	Self-absorbed
Musical	Odd facial expressions
'Sparky'	Clumsy
Confident	Learning difficulties
Sensitive	Distracted/hyperactive/impulsive
Sense of achievement	Testing boundaries; controlling/defiant

she videotaped, 12 behaved in slightly unexpected ways in the MTDA sessions. This is quite a large number if one considers that the research assistant had been working as a music therapist with this client group for a number of years and had experience of how children behaved in both group and individual music therapy sessions. This suggests that this group of children often behave differently in individual music therapy sessions and group sessions.

Her comments indicated that, in general, children often felt more relaxed in one-to-one sessions (MTDAs), were able to focus more easily and were more interactive. She mentioned several times that this might have been because group sessions were often difficult because of other children in the group who could be quite disturbed and disruptive. However, she felt that two of the children (C13 and C17) were less confident in the one-to-one sessions than in the group session.

Comments on the answers given by children in structured interviews

As indicated earlier in this chapter, it was not possible to interview all the children after their MTDA and ADOS assessments. Eighteen children were interviewed after both their MTDA and their ADOS sessions, a further seven children were interviewed after their MTDA sessions, one child was interviewed after his ADOS session, and four children were not interviewed at all.[*]

In what follows I make some general points and then comment on the results in both the MTDA and the ADOS questionnaires, taking each section of questions in the interview one at a time.

GENERAL COMMENTS

The general comments by the interviewer show that the children sometimes had difficulties remembering the ADOS test, whereas the MTDA session often immediately preceded the interview and was therefore easier to talk about. Sometimes children struggled to remain focused, particularly when being interviewed about the ADOS.

MOTIVATION/INTEREST

Generally, the children appeared to enjoy both MTDA and ADOS sessions. In many cases they could not identify anything in the tests they did not like. In the MTDA sessions, 9 out of 25 children were able to say they did not like one of the instruments, but they were all positive about some aspects of the session. In the ADOS sessions, 9 out of 19 children expressed a dislike for one or more of the activities, and three of those nine children had nothing positive to say about the sessions. It is interesting to note that out of the nine children who said they disliked one of the musical instruments in the MTDAs, three said that they disliked the instrument because it was too loud.

Most of the children were familiar with at least some aspects of both the ADOS and the MTDA tests. In the ADOS tests, out of the 14 children who answered this question, three were totally familiar with this type of test, four had done some of the activities before, and six felt all the material was new. In the MTDAs, out of the 24 children who answered this question, five felt very familiar with this type of session, 16 had played some of the instruments before, and three answered that they had never played any of the

*   Guidelines for the structured interviews with the children are included as Appendix 9.

instruments or games before. This was a little surprising for me, as I had expected children to be a lot more familiar with the ADOS types of test than with MTDA assessments.

EXPERIENCE OF BEING WITH ANOTHER PERSON

Again the responses of the children were mixed regarding how similar the sessions were to previous experiences. I was expecting the children to feed back that the MTDA sessions were more unfamiliar than the ADOS sessions, but this was not the case.

Nearly all the children said they enjoyed taking turns, in both tests. There were mixed responses when the children were asked whether they preferred choosing activities or having activities chosen for them. (This question was much more relevant in MTDA sessions than in ADOS sessions where the choices were all made by the tester.) In the MTDA, out of the 24 children who answered this question, twelve children preferred choosing themselves, seven preferred me choosing and five did not mind. In the ADOS, seven children answered the question; three would have preferred to choose if they could have done, four did not mind.

Almost all the children felt the ADOS and the MTDA tests were fun. About half the children questioned in each of the tests preferred playing alone, the other half preferred playing with the tester.

SELF-ESTEEM/CONFIDENCE

Many children needed prompting from the interviewer to help them to acknowledge that they were good at things or that it felt nice to be good at things. Out of a total of 37 questions asked about the MTDA in this section, 28 answers contained a positive element. Out of a total of 25 questions asked about the ADOS, 15 answers contained positive elements. This indicates that it may have been a little easier for children to acknowledge that they felt good about themselves in MTDA sessions than in ADOS sessions.

PERCEPTION OF ANOTHER PERSON'S FEELINGS

The children generally felt that the testers enjoyed the sessions in both MTDA and ADOS sessions. When asked about what the tester liked best in the MTDA sessions, out of 24 responses, 20 were definite and only four did not know. In the ADOS sessions, out of 18 responses, eight were definite and ten did not know. This is obviously an interesting finding and may reflect that in MTDA sessions, the tester is perhaps more actively involved with the children and more often playing as an equal. Although the tester also plays with the children in the ADOS, the role is that of an interested adult rather than that of a fellow musician.

Additional study comparisons

Autistc Diagnostic Interviews

As part of their treatment while they were at the Croft Unit, 23 out of the 30 experimental subjects had Autistic Diagnostic Interviews (ADIs). This assessment tool is very different from the MTDA or the ADOS because it consists of a detailed two- to three-hour interview with the parent of the child. There are three main sections to the test:

1. qualitative impairments in reciprocal social interaction

2. impairments in communication

3. repetitive behaviours and stereotyped patterns.

In order to be considered as either autistic or as having Asperger's syndrome, children have to score on or above the cut-off point for each of the three sections.

I have compared the results of the ADIs with those obtained from the MTDAs, the ADOS and the Croft diagnoses. However, I am aware that these comparisons are somewhat rough and must be considered with caution. This is because the ADI measures whether or not a child has autism or Asperger's syndrome whereas the other three methods of diagnosis are looking more broadly at whether or not a child is on the autistic spectrum.

Table 7.10 summarises the results of this comparison; more detailed results and tables are included in my PhD thesis (Oldfield 2004). Although 23 children had ADIs, one of these children was the same one whose ADOS could not be scored. This is why the columns with ADOS scores in them add up to 22 rather than 23.

This table shows that quite a high proportion of the ADI results disagree with the MTDA and the ADOS results. There is higher agreement, however, between the ADI and the Croft diagnosis. This could be an indication that the Croft diagnosis takes account of the opinions of the parents and the families of the children whereas the MTDA and the ADOS are purely assessing the child.

Comparison between MTDA-1 and MTDA-2

As explained in Chapter 2, the music therapy assessments at the Croft children's unit consist of two half-hour sessions, usually held with a weekly

Table 7.10 Summary of agreements and disagreements between the ADI and the other tests

	ADI and MTDA	ADI and ADOS	ADI and Croft	All four tests
Number of children where tests agree	14	12	18	8
Number of children where tests disagree	9	10	5	14

interval. When reflecting on the purpose of having two music therapy sessions rather than one, I came to the conclusion that the first session enabled me to get to know the child a little and helped the child to feel at ease in a somewhat unusual environment. It was in the second session that I felt I was able to assess the child's strengths and difficulties more effectively. This is why most of the data used in this project focuses on the second of the two MTDA sessions.

Nevertheless, during this research project, I did score the first of the two MTDA sessions as well as the second, so I can now compare the results of the scores in the sessions. As the sessions served different functions, I thought it would be interesting to see whether this would be reflected in different scores. When I was scoring, I was thinking purely in diagnostic terms rather than considering the first session as one that served mainly as a time to get to know the child.

The results are listed in my PhD thesis (Oldfield 2004) and were subjected to statistical analysis, showing that there was a significant difference between the scores in the two MTDAs. The mean of the second MTDA was slightly higher than the mean of the first MTDA, indicating that I was picking up more autistic-type characteristics in the second test. This result has clinical significance because it confirms that two rather than one MTDA are important for these children. If there had been no significant difference between the two sets of results then it might have been more difficult to justify the necessity of two MTDAs for each child.

Comparison between research assistant's and music therapist's MTDA results

When setting up this project I decided that it would be useful for the research assistant to videotaped as many of the MTDAs as possible. We used these videos to discuss children with the team at the Croft Unit and when we needed to check up on the results on the scoring sheets or on the testers' questionnaires. As the research assistant was present in the sessions she was able to fill in the MTDA scoring sheets independently from my scoring of the sessions. She was present for 26 of the 30 sessions, which means that we were able to compare our results for these 26 children.

The results were included in my PhD thesis (Oldfield 2004) and subjected to statistical analysis, indicating that there was no significant difference between our scores. This is very encouraging as it indicates that the test is giving similar results even when scored by independent music therapists.

Review of main findings in this chapter

The first important finding in the investigation described in this chapter was that the MTDA showed 72 per cent agreement with the ADOS regarding which diagnostic category a child was put into. This indicates that the new MTDA procedure was picking up similar information to the established and well-tried ADOS test.

Nevertheless, in addition, the MTDA and ADOS tests showed significant differences in their total scores. The two tests were clearly picking up different information on the children. The greatest number of disagreements between the two tests was with the borderline children.

The ADOS scores were significantly higher than the MTDA scores, indicating that, in general, the ADOS was picking up more autistic-type behaviours than the MTDA. When comparing individual questions within the MTDA and the ADOS tests, I found that there were only two sets of comparable categories that scored significantly differently: 'social overtures by the children' and 'ritualistic behaviours'. The MTDA was less likely to consider the children's social overtures to be autistic but more likely to score autistic-type behaviours when looking at the children's ritualistic behaviours.

In some ways this result ties in with the information gained from the children's structured interviews and the testers' questionnaires. The children's structured interviews indicated that the children felt slightly less inhibited and more at ease in MTDAs than in ADOS tests, but also at times more self-conscious. The testers' questionnaires indicated that ADOS testers placed more emphasis on spoken language whereas the MTDA testers were more interested in non-verbal communication. The ADOS testers looked more at social abilities and the MTDA tester at spontaneity. The MTDA sessions were less structured and more child-led than the ADOS tests and as a result children were perhaps slightly more at ease and less oppositional. However, the fact that the children were more spontaneous might have explained why they also displayed more ritualistic-type behaviours in the MTDA sessions.

It was encouraging to find that the children's structured interviews indicated that the children mostly thought that the MTDA and ADOS tests were fun. The testers themselves generally felt that they administered the test well. Both these findings make the two assessments appealing to use and user-friendly.

The reliability of the MTDA as an assessment tool was strengthened when I found that the music therapy research assistant's independent scoring of the sessions was not significantly different from my scoring.

The necessity for two as opposed to one MTDA test for each child was confirmed when I found that there was a significant difference between the first MTDA scores and the second MTDA scores: I was picking up more autistic behaviours in the second test. In addition the children's structured interviews and the testers' questionnaires indicated that a number of children were quite shy and self-conscious in MTDAs but often less so in the second MTDA session than in the first.

The other point that should be considered is that this research project investigated a new diagnostic assessment by looking at mostly borderline children rather than including a cross-section of children, which would include a higher proportion of 'normal' children and 'classically autistic' children who are easier to diagnose. In other words the MTDA was put to the test with those children who are hardest to diagnose. As the MTDA has given us useful information even with the most difficult group of children to diagnose, it would indicate that the MTDA could be a valuable diagnostic tool for psychiatric teams to include in their assessment packages.

The hypothesis put forward at the beginning of this investigation was that the MTDAs were effective at highlighting important aspects of behaviour which are symptomatic of (or exclude) a diagnosis of autistic spectrum disorder. In many ways this hypothesis has been shown to be correct. Nevertheless, the number of children assessed was too small for there to be significant differences in many of the sub-categories of the MTDAs and the ADOS tests.

The findings in this chapter have many possible implications for the future of MTDAs both at the Croft and for other music therapists. In the future I hope to look into how to train other music therapists to use MTDAs in other child and family psychiatric units. However, further research looking at larger numbers of children would be needed to firmly establish the MTDA as a reliable assessment tool.

Another area that would be interesting to explore would be to look at applying MTDAs to other client groups, either younger or older children with possible autistic spectrum disorders or children with other possible psychiatric disorders such as attention deficit disorder, attachment disorders or specific language disorders. In a companion book (Oldfield 2006) I describe research investigating individual music therapy treatment with ten preschool children with autistic spectrum disorder and their parents. Many of the parents were surprised at how quickly their children had become engaged in the initial music therapy assessment sessions. This would indicate that a non-verbal, but potentially very motivating, assessment procedure such as the MTDA could be of value with this age group.

Chapter 8

Teaching Music Therapy

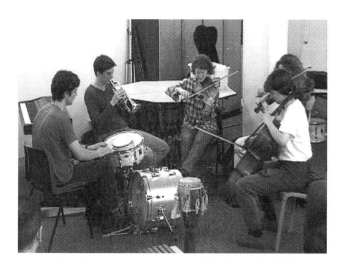

Introduction

This chapter focuses on informing other people about music therapy and passing on music therapy skills.

Nearly all music therapists are asked to give talks or workshops on various aspects of music therapy, either within the clinical settings or to groups of people interested in music therapy, such as parent groups or charities such as the National Autistic Society or Mencap. I shall start by describing a basic structure for a workshop that I have found works well. I then go on to describe some aspects of my work at Anglia Ruskin University (previously Anglia Polytechnic University or APU) where I have been working as a lecturer on the MA in music therapy training course for the past 11 years. Finally I write about the process of making music therapy training videos.

Music therapy workshops

Music therapists are constantly asked to explain what they do. Usually I enjoy answering questions about my work and have various answers that I use frequently, often referring to on-going clinical work without revealing names or personal details. Occasionally, when I am very tired and people ask me what I do I wish I could reply 'computer analyst' or 'plumber', for example, as I might then not have to give lengthy explanations. This happens particularly when people say 'Really, music therapy! How fascinating, but does it actually work?' My answer is usually something along the lines of: 'Yes, I often get through to children and families by music making, and can help in various ways.' At times, however, I have been very tempted to respond: 'No it doesn't work, but I have enjoyed getting paid for trying for the past 25 years.'

When I am asked to do a general introduction about music therapy and half an hour or more is available, I nearly always suggest that it would be beneficial to include some practical components where participants (or at least some of the participants if the group is too large) are involved in playing simple percussion or wind instruments.

The content of music therapy workshops depends on the background and experience of the people who are attending, the number of people present, the purpose of the session, the time available, the place where the workshop is being held and what equipment is available. Over the years I have found that I have a general format I adapt to suit different circumstances and needs. The clinical examples and video excerpts I choose will be selected to illustrate the clinical specialities and interests of the group participants.

The following is a description of a 'standard' workshop on music therapy that I ran recently. The workshop lasted one and a half hours and took place at the Croft Unit for Child and Family Psychiatry as part of an open day which aimed to inform other professionals and interested people about the work on the unit.

I ran the group in the Croft music therapy room and because of the size of the room I could accommodate only 12 people at a time. I repeated the workshop later in the day so that another group of 12 people could attend.

I placed the chairs in a circle and explained that I would do some talking, we would then experiment with playing some of the instruments and I would conclude the workshop by showing some video excerpts of music therapy sessions. I said that participants should feel free to ask questions throughout the workshop and that the exploratory playing of instruments would be to illustrate points about music therapy rather than a chance to explore personal feelings through playing in great depth.

I started the workshop by explaining that I have worked as a music therapist for 25 years and presently work at the Croft Unit for Child and Family Psychiatry, the Child Development Centre and at Anglia Ruskin University where I am involved in training music therapists.

I explained how music therapists are trained in the UK, emphasising that music therapy training is at a postgraduate level and that music therapists are usually musicians first and then train to apply their musical skills in a clinical setting. I outlined the different clinical areas that music therapists work in, making it clear that although my work has been mainly with children and families many other music therapists work with adults in a wide range of settings.

I then defined music therapy, outlining the fact that music therapists use music as a means to an end. I gave a clinical example of a child with Asperger's syndrome who usually spoke in a stilted way and struggled to make conversations flow; she was drawn into improvised and spontaneous non-verbal musical turn-taking. The aim, which was to increase spontaneity in communication, was non-musical. The means, which was an improvised exchange between the child playing percussion instruments and the therapist on the piano, was musical.

This talking took about 10–15 minutes, after which I suggested that we should do some playing. I explained that I would be illustrating what I felt were the main reasons why music therapy worked through our playing. The aspects I focused on were motivation, play, structure and control, but I did not tell the group that these were the areas I was demonstrating until after we had done each of the four practical activities.

Motivation

I invited the participants to stand up and choose a musical instrument from a wide selection of percussion, string and wind instruments stored in a very large cupboard along the wall on one side of the room. I told the group to experiment with various instruments, taking their time to try them out and explore different sounds. While people were choosing I stood near the cupboard answering questions about how individual instruments were played, what they were called and where they came from. Once everyone had chosen an instrument and sat down with the instrument on their lap or in front of them I sat at the piano and when everyone was ready said very clearly 'Let's all play together' before starting to play myself.

I played an energetic, engaging tune that was easy to follow rhythmically and harmonically. As I played I turned towards the group, obviously interacting musically with participants. Once everybody was playing with me and secure rhythmically, I slowed down and then changed from 4/4 to 3/4. I then speeded up again and played randomly all over the keyboard, in a free and chaotic way. Finally I came back to the familiar tune of 'What Shall We Do with a Drunken Sailor?' and played this several times before making a very clear ending. During my playing, each time I changed my rhythm or style I waited for the group to follow me before making the next change.

When I finished the playing I left a dramatic silence for a few seconds and then said that what we had just done was one of the principal reasons why I felt music therapy was effective. I went on to explain that without me having to say anything, the group had instinctively followed my changes of tempi, my changes of dynamic and my changes of style. Nobody had consciously analysed the music making process and yet we had all played together in a cohesive way, listening and following one another. The rhythms and the clear harmonic phrases had motivated everyone to play and take part. This drive to be part of the group music making was present in very young babies, people with severe learning disabilities and people with Alzheimer's disease, amongst others.

Play

I selected a large drum and a cymbal on a stand and put these two instruments in front of me. I had a hard and loud beater for the drum in one hand, and a soft and quiet beater for the cymbal in my other hand. I told the group that the idea of the game was for individual people in the group to charm me into relinquishing my seat and my instruments, by playing their instruments to me in such an engaging way that I could not resist changing places with whoever had gained my attention. The game was non-verbal but I would play the drum to indicate that 'no, I was not going to change places' or the cymbal when I was beginning to hesitate. Before getting up I would play the cymbal to indicate 'yes, you can have my seat'. Once another person had gained my place it was his or her turn to play the drum and the cymbal while the rest of the group tried to gain the drummer's interest and be allowed to take that place. Quickly the group realised that it was more effective to wait for a pause and then play while looking clearly at the drum player. Non-verbal facial expression was important, and there was lots of laughter as some drummers clearly refused to let others play, or were finally charmed by persistent or distinctive sounds, and confirmed their intention to change places through soft cymbal sounds.

After several people had had a turn on the drum and the cymbal I brought the activity to an end. I explained that this game had shown that musical interactions were a good and easy way to enable people to exchange and play in a non-verbal way. People were quickly able to be humorous and have fun together. I went on to say that this aspect of music making was particularly valuable when working with parents who struggled to be playful with their children or children who had communication difficulties when using language.

Structure

I asked the group to put their instruments down on the floor and to stand up. I clapped four times in a steady crotchet = 120 in 4/4 and indicated to the group that they should imitate and echo back my clapping. I then varied my clapping rhythms but continued to keep to the 4/4 pulse. When I felt that the rhythms I was clapping were becoming hard to imitate I would insert another bar of four crotchets that were very straightforward to copy. I then, gradually, started adding vocal sounds and movements to my 4/4 clapping units, at first stamping and adding 'boo' sounds and then twirling on the spot or jumping with glissando vocal sounds or loud shouts to accompany my movements. I then encouraged someone else to lead and to pass on this leadership to another group member once they felt they had had enough of suggesting rhythms to the others.

Once several people had had a turn leading I explained to the group that this exchange very clearly demonstrated how music occurred in time and how we were reassured by familiar and predictable rhythms. The fact that the leader was clapping a rhythm within an expected and straightforward 4/4 rhythm enabled the group to echo back the sound with confidence and ease. I indicated that the use of rhythm and structure was central to my work, both when interacting with a child through improvised musical exchanges and to organise the session and have reassuring and predictable beginnings and endings of sessions.

Control

I made sure we had the same numbers of chairs as participants with no empty chairs left in the room and invited everyone to choose an instrument. I sat at the piano and before starting to play explained that I would lead from the piano and we would all play together. When the piano stopped we would all leave our instruments and move to another chair. What this meant was that after I had finished playing the piano someone else would end up at the piano as the leader of the group. In my initial turn on the piano I made sure that I incorporated some random rhythmical playing as well as a tune such as 'Three Blind Mice', played with one finger, in order to reassure the group that any kind of piano playing was acceptable.

After four group participants had played the piano I brought the activity to a close and explained that this experience showed that it was very easy to switch leaders in group music playing. In my clinical work, I could therefore very easily address issues of control in music therapy groups and sessions. This is important because so many difficulties that children and families experience in child and family psychiatry are linked to not feeling in control, or taking too much control.

Cases

After the group musical interactions I briefly presented two cases showing excerpts from music therapy sessions on video. The first case was a music therapy diagnostic assessment with a boy who was subsequently diagnosed as having Asperger's syndrome. The second was a family music therapy session with a mother, a father, a boy of seven with attention deficit syndrome and his little sister aged four. This family was struggling to manage both children and the music therapy sessions provided one of the few moments in the week when they were all able to relax and have fun together. In both cases I tried, on the one hand, to highlight in what way music therapy was different from other groups and approaches on the unit. On the other hand, I explained how music therapy fitted into the unit's general assessment and treatment programmes. I also again highlighted the importance of motivation, play, structure and control in the sessions, linking my clinical music therapy work with the group participants' recent practical experience.

Questions and discussions

The last ten minutes of the workshop were devoted to questions and discussions. There was a question on whether there were musical activities I could suggest that could be used by other staff with groups of children. I suggested various books and tapes, but also explained that much of my work was dependent on spontaneous improvisation and music making and would be difficult to do without special training. Another question concerned the general availability of music therapists in the area. I explained that in addition to myself working at the Croft and at the Child Development Centre, there was a team of music therapists working in special and mainstream schools in and around Cambridge. One of the group participants' commented that she would have liked to play the instruments for longer. She said that she had taken a little time to feel at ease and just as she was really getting into it I brought the playing to an end. I answered that if more time had been available it might have been possible to explore participants' music making further and to focus in more depth on the experience of playing together. I explained that this particular workshop was more of a teaching session than an in-depth exploratory music making session.

The general feedback from participants in the two workshops was excellent. The two aspects that participants had felt were particularly useful were the clinical examples on video and the experience of practical music making. Many people said that they had been nervous to start with but had then had great fun. Several people said that the playing had been the highlight of their day.

As a music therapist, I think it is very important to run regular workshops for staff and others who may be interested in the work. Unless people have experienced group music making it is very easy to have misconceptions about how the music therapist either teaches children and families to sing or play an instrument, or simply plays music for people to listen to. If staff have felt what it is like to play music in a group they will have a much clearer idea who might benefit from music therapy and why it is an invaluable way of working with children and families.

Training music therapists

The music therapy MA at Anglia Ruskin University

In the late 1980s and the early 1990s my music therapy colleague, Helen Odell-Miller, and I started discussing the idea of setting up a local music therapy course. We knew there was a need for a course outside London and had ideas about what we felt would be useful to include. Having both worked for over ten years in the National Health Service we felt that music therapy trainees would benefit from being immersed in clinical settings in block placements in a similar way to nurses in training. We also realised that the multi-disciplinary teams we worked in would have a lot to offer music therapy trainees. We knew we each had different approaches to our music therapy work, which was partly due to the fact that Helen worked in adult psychiatry and I worked with children and families. But we felt this would be an asset for students rather than a disadvantage. We wanted to create a training course where students learnt about several music therapy approaches in great depth, and were introduced to a number of other methods. Then, depending on the setting the students worked in and their own particular strengths and preferences they would ultimately make up their own minds about which way they would each choose to work, developing and adapting approaches as necessary.

The music department at Anglia Ruskin University in Cambridge (previously Anglia Polytechnic University) was very interested in the idea of setting up a music therapy training course. Our first postgraduate music therapy MA course started in September 1994 after many months of meetings and planning. Initially, the course lasted one year at which point students gained a music therapy diploma allowing them to work as a music therapist. They then had the option to complete an MA dissertation within six years of starting training. It is anticipated that from September 2006, the course will last two years, including the MA dissertation.

Since 1994, I have been teaching music therapy students on this course. There are many aspects of this work and of the course in general that could be described and written about. More information about the content of the course and the admissions procedure can be obtained from the Anglia Ruskin University music department. In 1999, I made a training video about the course which we use on open days or when we are giving presentations about the training (Oldfield *et al.* 1999). Here I shall focus on three aspects of training that I feel are particularly important, and that are closely linked to the interactive music therapy approach I describe in this and in my companion book (Oldfield 2006). These are: my general teaching philosophy; teaching single-line improvisation; and teaching students on clinical placements.

My general teaching philosophy

For the past 11 years I have been involved in training music therapists on our MA course. I have discovered that I really enjoy this work. There are four points that I believe are particularly important in my teaching.

REMAINING CLOSE TO CLINICAL PRACTICE

In my teaching, I have always remained very close to my weekly clinical musical practice, continually referring to cases I am currently treating and situations that arise in the clinical teams. I use video excerpts of music therapy sessions to demonstrate theoretical points, and the clinical material brings the theory to life and is of immediate relevance to students. As I am involved in a clinical music therapy process myself, I know the client and the music therapy processes I am referring to intimately, and can speak with confidence, enthusiasm and passion. The students' comments and questions will allow me to reflect on my on-going clinical work, which will help me to define and describe my particular music therapy approach.

BUILDING ON EXISTING STRENGTHS

It is important for students to gain a wide range of knowledge regarding how a variety of music therapists work in different clinical settings. Nevertheless, it is equally important for students to learn to understand their own strengths and difficulties, both musically and clinically. Once confidence is acquired in one or two improvisational styles with a specific client group, for example, students will be ready to expand this expertise and work on the areas they find more difficult. My approach is to quickly identify students' individual strengths and give positive feedback and encouragement. I emphasise that all music therapists have different areas of skills and am open about my own strengths and weaknesses. Once students have gained initial confidence, I will be open and honest about work that needs to be done to improve weaknesses, while continuing to be encouraging and positive about individual student's strengths.

CONTINUING TO BE INSPIRED BY MUSIC OR MUSIC MAKING

As a music therapist my principal way of relating to people is through music making. In order to ensure that the way I play, improvise and listen to music remains creative and alive it is important to continuously explore, nurture and understand my own passion for music and to encourage the students to do this. The particular musical interest or passion to be nurtured may vary from student to student, depending on what instruments they play and which musical styles they are experienced and proficient in. As a lecturer I encourage students to remain in touch with their own excitement and enthusiasm for music. I try to encourage students to nurture, value and pursue their own interest in music making.

A BALANCED METHOD OF DELIVERY

I always present lectures and workshops in a varied way, balancing talking with showing video excerpts of clinical work and demonstrating points through involving the students in active music making. I make use of overheads and Microsoft PowerPoint but also talk freely, often referring to clients I am currently working with. I try to have a clear structure and shape to my teaching sessions, but also allow myself to be drawn into debates that arise from questions asked, and reflect with the students in creative ways.

Single-line instrumental improvisation

In Oldfield (2006) I explain how I use my clarinet in almost all my music therapy sessions. There are several reasons why single-line instruments are invaluable in music therapy. The most important of these is that, if the instrument we are most proficient on is a single-line instrument, we are likely to be able to communicate most effectively by playing it.

I also talked about the advantages of alternating singing with single-line instrument playing and the importance of being able to move around the room while playing. Being mobile enables the music therapist to be playful, at times running away and at other times looking directly at clients.

Single-line instruments allow us to vary the pitches and dynamics on individual notes and easily incorporate silences into the playing. The way individual notes are started and ended will be important and may effect the overall shapes of improvisations.

For all these reasons it is important for students – and particularly those whose first study is a single-line instrument – to learn to improvise with confidence on that instrument in the clinical situation. I teach students single-line clinical improvisation in small groups of around six or seven. In our first session I try to enable the students to play freely and explore, without being concerned about how good they are, or getting it 'right'. This is sometimes quite difficult, particularly for classically trained orchestral players who may have spent many years striving for perfection. I also address practical issues such as: when to take instruments out of cases in sessions; tuning instruments, wetting reeds or warming up instruments before sessions; deciding whether or not clients are allowed to play the therapist's instrument; and having a safe place within the room where the instrument can be put down quickly and safely.

By the second session I will be encouraging students to practise improvising in pairs, focusing on both creating a quiet relaxed atmosphere and, as a contrast, playing in energetic and fast ways. I will suggest to students that they should start to identify what aspects of improvising they find easy and what aspects they find difficult. Some students, for example, are very good at meandering in an engaging jazzy style but find it difficult to give the overall improvisation a convincing structure or shape. Others are very strong rhythmically but struggle to play in a convincing tonality. I also suggest to students that they should look out for their own and their improvisation partner's musical characteristics. They should allow themselves to revel in those aspects of playing that they particularly enjoy and then see whether they can experiment with taking on their partner's characteristic ways of playing.

Depending on what aspects students need help with I might suggest improvising in pentatonic or modal scales. Sometimes we use a three-note leitmotif to come back to, or I will suggest alternating between a clear four- or eight-bar rhythmic phrase and a rhythmically free passage. By the third session students will improvise individually within the group, with another student pretending to be the client and playing the drum or the wind chimes. When a particular improvisation is very effective I encourage the group to reflect on why this is the case, what was special about the music, the way the student played or the body language used.

By the second or third session I usually start encouraging students to use their voice in conjunction with their instrument. Some students find either the instrumental improvisations or the use of the voice much easier, so I encourage these students to use whichever they find easier as a supportive tool for the thing they find more difficult. I also suggest that students should incorporate silences into their improvisations, experimenting with different lengths of silence and exploring silences that feel calm and relaxed, and silences that feel uncomfortable and create tension.

We then start adding movement and drama. I continue to encourage students to work in pairs, changing partners every week and then performing in pairs in our weekly sessions. As sessions progress the students get to know each others' musical characteristics. Some students will work on very specific issues such as making sure they look at clients while they are playing. For others, the work will focus on more complex issues such as creating a good balance between structure and freedom or alternating between listening to and taking on the clients' musical ideas and initiating their own.

During these teaching sessions I have to get to know each student's specific way of playing and identify some strengths and weaknesses in their improvisations. Although I do try to help students overcome their difficulties I am also very positive and encouraging and help the students to get in touch with how much fun it is to improvise and develop their own individual styles of playing. In my experience, the most important aspect of teaching single-line improvisation skills is to develop the students' confidence and belief in their own abilities.

Teaching students on clinical placements

For the past 20 years, I have regularly had students on clinical placement with me. I have always found the experience of students shadowing my work as a music therapist challenging, stimulating and very rewarding. From 1994 onwards, the students who have been on placement with me have all come from the music therapy MA at Anglia Ruskin University. Before 1994, students came from the Guildhall School of Music and Drama, from the Roehampton Institute and from music therapy training courses in Denmark, Germany and Australia. Over ten years ago, I wrote some preliminary observations on teaching music therapy students on practical placements (Oldfield 1992). Some of the comments in this section are similar to the thoughts expressed in that article.

Clinical placements are possibly the most important part of a music therapist's training. Although theories about music therapy are emerging and there has been a recent increase in books written by music therapists, music therapy remains a very practical profession. Most music therapists would agree that they have learnt and developed largely through clinical experience, acquiring new skills and expertise each time they are confronted with new clinical situations.

It is difficult to generalise about how students learn on clinical placements because each will not only have different strengths, skills and experience but will find certain ways of learning easier than others. In addition, essential skills such as clinical improvisation are difficult to describe and define precisely as so much is dependent on the personality of the therapist, the musical preferences and general profile of each individual client, the inspiration of the moment and the therapist's intuition.

In my role as placement supervisor I try to provide students with opportunities to observe and experience music therapy in practice. I will initially encourage students to gain an understanding of how music therapy fits into the clinical setting and the role music therapy plays within the multi-disciplinary team. The students also need to understand the reasons why clients are referred both to the clinic and to music therapy, and what types of difficulty the clients are experiencing. I try to give the students written information about the clinical settings as well as copies of articles and handouts that are relevant to the clinical work so that I do not have to give this information verbally. This allows the focus of our work to be on the students' practical experience, rather than on my imparting knowledge to them. As well as acquiring knowledge, the students need to gain confidence to feel relaxed and at ease within the clinical setting. Students are usually nervous about their first music therapy sessions. There may be an underlying fear about whether or not they will be able to improvise musically with clients or generally whether they can be 'good enough' therapists. One of my most important tasks is therefore to gain the students' trust so that they can relax sufficiently to develop their own confidence.

When a student observes my music therapy sessions, I try to explain about each client briefly before the session. I ask the student to sit quietly in a corner of the room, if necessary pretending to read a book if the client seems to be aware of being observed. Of course I ask my clients and their parents whether they will mind being observed, and if I feel that having the student in the room will be in any way disruptive or intrusive the student will not come in. In most cases, however, students will be able to observe my work directly. I feel this is important because students learn a huge amount from being in the room with me and my clients, and I often gain new insights into the work I am doing from discussing the work with the students after sessions.

When students first start their own clinical music therapy work on the placements, the difficulties they experience usually centre around two interconnected aspects of the work. These are developing a relationship with the clients, and clinical improvisation. They also have to develop group techniques and learn to fit into a team.

DEVELOPING A RELATIONSHIP WITH THE CLIENT

Students who have been accepted on to music therapy training courses in the UK will have been judged to have the ability to form relationships with a wide variety of clients. Many students will have already worked with people with learning difficulties or psychiatric disorders, but some will have had experience in only one of the many areas in which music therapists work. The very first hurdle that some students have to overcome is that of getting used to working with very disabled or aggressive young children or dysfunctional families with severally emotionally disturbed children. This may cause the student a great deal of anxiety and it is important to support the student during this period and to explain that it is quite normal to be ill at ease or uncomfortable with some clients at first. This does not mean that the student is insensitive and is unsuitable to be a music therapist. Gradually, as the student gets to know individual clients and groups of clients this unease will disappear, often to the extent that at the end of the placement the student finds it difficult to remember ever having felt ill at ease.

In the same way some students will be shy about helping very fragile or severely physically disabled children. I might have to spend time physically helping such clients in front of the student in order to allay these fears.

Another difficulty that some students experience when working with very young children is that of being overwhelmed by how appealing or sweet the toddlers look when they are playing the instruments. While I think it can be helpful to be charmed by engaging children and through this process to be drawn into creative musical exchanges, it is also important to remember the overall therapeutic objectives and remind oneself what the purpose of the work is.

Some students I have worked with have struggled not to become over-involved with the children and families they have been treating. At times the students have become upset and angry about all the difficulties a family may have experienced and end up finding fault with all the other people caring for the family. These students may need to assess whether their own emotions and feelings are getting in the way. If unresolved difficulties arise for the students, I sometimes suggest that they might want to explore these feelings further in their own regular personal therapy (which is a compulsory part of the training). It is also important to explain that the student must not let the child split the clinical team. Underlying conflicts between different professionals involved with the family usually harm, rather than help, the client.

Once the student can feel at ease with a client and can avoid either over-identifying or feeling sorry for the client, the student can attempt to steer the relationship with the client in a particular direction. Initial sessions will probably include exploratory work on a variety of instruments, and the student will gradually get to know the client musically as well as generally. Developing a musical relationship with a client will include discovering a client's musical preferences or abilities. This may involve finding out about a child's general preferences regarding certain songs or a specific style of music, or discovering that a client particularly responds to certain pitches, rhythms, tone colours or volume. It should be a two-way process between the child and the student. The two people find common musical ground that will enable them to develop a relationship and communicate.

CLINICAL IMPROVISATION

All students will have passed an instrumental audition and some will have taken part in an assessed group improvisation before starting their training. They will have shown that they are able to improvise musically on one or two instruments, or at least that they have the potential to learn to improvise fairly quickly and easily.

Many students find, however, that once they are in the clinical situation, the instrument on which they are the most competent is not the one that they want to use all the time. Second-study piano students often feel that they want to develop their piano improvisation skills, as this tends to be a very useful instrument for holding the attention of a group of people or for steering a group improvisation in one direction or another. First-study piano students, on the other hand, who lack confidence on their second instrument, are stuck when faced with a situation where no piano is available, or when it is necessary to be close to a client (on the floor, for example) and the piano is not suitable.

A large proportion of students experience difficulties at first when using their voice to sing and improvise. Trained singers sometimes struggle because their training teaches them to prepare their voices and to concentrate fully on the quality of the sound they are going to produce, making it difficult for them to react vocally to the client in a spontaneous way. Untrained singers may be shy about using their voice and need help and encouragement to experiment and develop their skills.

Whatever their first or second instruments, most students need to develop confidence in their spontaneous use of musical improvisation. Even the most skilled musical improvisers worry at times about whether they should play in one key or another, whether they should use tonal or atonal improvisation, or whether they should improvise around a given tune rather than inventing completely new material. Students who are not so skilled in musical improvisation worry about repeating the same harmonies or tunes, about harmonic 'mistakes', or about being unable to play a given tune by ear without the odd wrong note. In fact all students need to develop their own style of clinical musical improvisation and build on the areas in which they feel strong. It is more important for the music to come out spontaneously and with confidence than for the musical improvisation to be a work of art in itself. In many cases the simpler types of musical response are by far the most effective. There are times when students do need to work on the actual technique of an instrument, and on extending their musical repertoire on an instrument, before they can develop the confidence which will lead to effective spontaneous improvisation. In most cases, however, the skills are there and it is simply a question of developing the necessary confidence. In my experience, students who truly love playing an instrument (even if it is not their first instrument) usually develop the ability to respond musically with confidence quite quickly.

I think it is also important not to forget that the student's confidence may be influenced by whether or not he or she feels able to do what the supervisor is doing in the clinical situation. As the supervisor may play totally different instruments and have very different musical strengths from those of the student, this may leave the student feeling inadequate when in fact it is more important to develop the student's personal skills rather than trying to copy the supervisor.

Once they have developed some confidence, many students find it relatively easy to follow clients musically and to respond to what the client is offering. They find it much more difficult, however, when a client offers little or no musical contributions, or when a client is very obstructive. When a client is interacting musically, students often do not know what to do with this musical dialogue, struggling to take on a leading role and steering the interaction in a particular direction. One answer to these difficulties is for the student to reflect on what the clinical improvisation is for, and in exactly what way he or she is trying to help the client. Although initial music therapy sessions may be mainly exploratory, the student must be clear, even in early sessions, about what issues are being explored and what questions are being asked. As treatment progresses the student should have specific aims and objectives and must be quite clear what these goals are. This clarity will help give the student's clinical improvisation a focus and a specific purpose. The student will then know, for example, whether the client will benefit from simply being supported and accompanied in the musical improvisation, or whether the student needs to improvise in a more intrusive way to enable changes to occur. Whatever the student decides upon, it is important to know which approach is being taken and why this choice has been made. The clinical improvisations then have a clear purpose and the student usually no longer feels stuck about what to do next.

A number of students experience difficulties with the flow and timing of their improvisations, particularly if the client's responses are erratic. Some students are so anxious to pick up every single cue from a client, to follow every movement a client makes, that they end up providing very interrupted and scattered music which then reinforces the disjointed behaviour the client is showing. In this case, students need encouragement to structure and round off improvisations that have been started, and at times to have the confidence to stick to whatever musical idea they have begun even if the client has dashed off in another direction. There may also be ways of both providing musical continuity and following the client. For example, if an improvisation has been started on a wind instrument and the client shows signs of losing interest, the therapist can regain attention by singing the client's name using the same style of melody in order not to interrupt the flow of the music.

DEVELOPING GROUP TECHNIQUES

There are a number of things that students may need to consider when working with groups of people rather than individuals. These include looking directly at all group members, waiting for silences before giving verbal or musical instructions, giving clear and simple messages, and planning activities within a group so that the desired balance between attention to individuals and attention to the group as a whole is achieved. There is no set pattern for pacing group sessions and in most cases the therapist will have to take the lead from group participants before or during the session. Again, however, the student needs to be clear what the therapeutic goals are for individual clients within the group. It will also help develop the student's confidence to prepare and plan group sessions even if the plans are not adhered to and other ideas seem more appropriate as the session develops.

When working with groups, the student needs to be aware not only of the relationship the student has with the client but also of the relationship between the clients, between the clients and the other staff in the group, and between the staff (including the student) working within the group. The sympathies and tensions between group members can often be used to develop therapeutic aims. So, for example, an angry child may be asked to thump, kick or head-butt a series of cushions while the member of staff towards whom the anger was directed accompanies the blows with different instruments. Clients who are intimidated by other, more extrovert group members may be asked to distribute instruments and possibly conduct an improvisation. In both cases, the relationships within the group determine the way in which music will be used within the group, and students must therefore be aware of the relationships within the group as well as being flexible about the planning about activities for the group.

LEARNING TO FIT INTO A TEAM

Many students start out with unrealistic ideas about how they would like to work and may at first find it difficult to compromise. They may, for example, be unwilling to push or even persuade a reluctant client to attend a session, and take no notice of the fact that experienced staff, who know the client well, suggest that once the first few difficult moments are over the client usually benefits from individual help offered. Some students may insist on using their own approach even if it is contrary to that of the institution they are working in. Such students may choose to be directive when the general philosophy of the centre is a very open approach, or (more commonly) to give no direction whatsoever to a client when the general approach is a more directive one. A student's strong, and often idealistic, views should not be ignored, because the supervisor can learn from these approaches and should always be willing to question and sometimes to challenge established ways of working. However, radical views which go against the general way in which a centre works must be treated with caution. To begin with, such approaches must be discussed with other staff, who should be happy about 'new' ideas being tried out. Thought must always be given to the fact that the client may be confused by a radically different way of working, and that a student's placements may not be long enough to warrant the disruption caused to the client and the centre. In general, a student will probably learn more by adapting and fitting in with the way in which the institution works, even if the student ultimately chooses to work in a different way.

Students also need to learn how to communicate in the best possible way with other staff involved with the same clients. Written or verbal reports may need to be short and simple to be read and understood. In many cases an informal discussion with a member of staff at the right moment may be far more valuable than a lengthy report written much later. Students often struggle with the fact that, although detailed analyses of sessions are valuable and important, there is often not enough time to do this in the clinical situation. In college, the student will have as much time as is needed to think about cases in great depth. In the clinical situation, however, the student will have to come to terms with compromise and be able to adapt to a wide variety of different teams and philosophical outlooks.

Making music therapy training videos

However intense a music therapy experience is, once it is over one has to rely on one's memory to recreate or remember the event. Unlike a painting which provides tangible evidence of an artistic creation, a musical performance or improvisation cannot be handled or visually examined. For the music therapist, this ephemeral nature of music can be an advantage as it may allow a client freedom of expression without feeling that there will be recorded tangible evidence of the experience. The disadvantage is that the therapist has to rely entirely on memory to analyse the work that has been done.

Audio or video recordings of music therapy sessions change this situation as it becomes possible to look back on the event and reflect and relive processes that occurred. In this book and in Oldfield (2006) I have explained how the use of videotapes can be helpful to children and families in sessions; I have also written about how useful micro-analyses of video-tapes can be in research investigations. In this section I shall describe the training videos I have made, and in what ways they have been useful.

One of the principal reasons why I felt that it was important to put together training videos was in order to provide information about music therapy without having to be present myself. When I started work in Cambridge in the early 1980s, I was one of only two music therapists in the area and was very frequently asked to run workshops for local hospitals or special schools. Unfortunately it was not always possible to spare the time to run workshops, particularly when it meant travelling long distances. The video excerpts I showed of my clinical work always seemed to be one of the most important and easiest ways to explain what I was doing, so it seemed logical to try to put these excerpts together and create a teaching tool. Before filming clients I would always gain verbal and written consent to do so. When making training videos I would again obtain verbal and written consent about the use of filmed excerpts. Even if written consent was given, I would not automatically use the material. If I felt in any way uncomfortable about a particular excerpt, or had any doubts in my mind that a client or a member of the family was not completely at ease with the material I was using, I would either discuss it with them again or not use that material.

The process of choosing excerpts and writing a script for the voiceover that would link these excerpts helped me to reflect on the methods I was using in my work. For my first training video, Richard Cramp, who at the time worked in the medical photography department at Addenbrookes Hospital, videotaped music therapy sessions at the Child Development Centre and we edited the videos together. I soon learnt that the process was long and at times required huge amounts of patience, but that there was no point in being frustrated when cables could not be found, or machines did not work. I also quickly realised that it was imperative that I came to our editing sessions with very clear ideas about which excerpts I wanted and exactly which frame I wanted to start and end the excerpt with.

My first training video about music therapy at the Child Development Centre was completed in 1992 (Oldfield and Cramp 1992) and was the first available in the UK to the general public for purchase. I received enthusiastic feedback from non-music therapists who wanted to find out about music therapy, but some more dubious feedback from other music therapists who were concerned that this audiovisual document would mean that all would be expected to work as I did. In some ways I can see that this was an understandable reaction to the first public training video. However, I also think that music therapists in general, but particularly those who feel they have very different or specific ways of working, should be spurred on to make their own videos so that a richer and more complete picture of music therapy practice is available to all.

Since 1992, I have made five more music therapy training videos and sold over 700 copies (Oldfield and Cramp 1994; Oldfield, MacDonald and Nudds 1999; Oldfield, MacDonald and Nudds 2000; Oldfield and Nudds 2002; Oldfield and Nudds 2005). Since I started working at Anglia Ruskin University in 1994, I have been making videos with the university media production department and their professional expertise has meant that two of the videos have won Royal Television Society Awards. I have continued to very much enjoy the whole process of making videos and still find I learn about my work through putting the films together. The music therapy profession in the UK has grown used to my videos and I now receive very positive feedback from my colleagues. I hope that in the future many other music therapists will make training videos about their work.

Conclusion

Apart from practising as a music therapist the other aspects of my work that I enjoy most of all are talking about my work and training music therapy students. As a university lecturer on the music therapy MA training course I am very fortunate to always be teaching mature, intelligent students who are highly motivated and interested. My clinical work forms the basis of my teaching, and the students' questions and feedback make me think about and improve my music therapy practice.

Chapter 9

Music Therapy Supervision

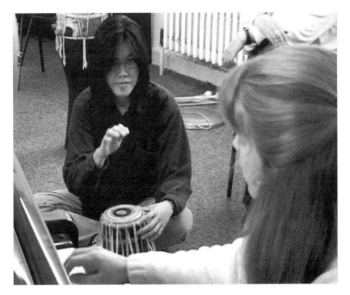

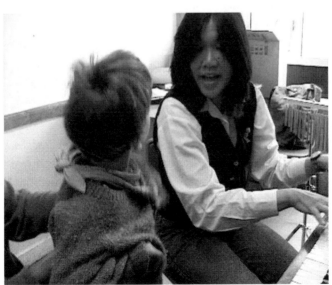

Introduction

In the early 1980s when I started working as a music therapist, it was not usual to have or give clinical supervision. At the time I shared an office with a speech therapist and the clinical psychologist, Malcolm Adams, who has helped me with all my research, worked in the next-door office. We provided informal but invaluable support for one another on an almost daily basis and in many ways this support system made up for the fact that we did not have formal clinical supervision sessions.

Twenty-five years later it has become a statutory requirement for newly qualified music therapists to have clinical supervision. Most employers pay for at least some supervision for their therapists, and the majority of music therapists make on-going arrangements for clinical supervision even once they have become experienced clinicians. I have found the experience of receiving clinical supervision invaluable, have very much enjoyed giving it and cannot now imagine not having or not giving supervision. However, I wonder whether the fact that we did not have formal clinical supervision in the early 1980s, in some ways made us work more closely together and contributed to the strong multi-disciplinary team.

I began having formal monthly clinical supervision when I started working in child and family psychiatry, in 1987. A few years later, in 1990, I became an Association of Professional Music Therapists(APMT) clinical supervisor and started supervising other music therapists on an individual basis. Between September 2000 and July 2003, I ran a clinical supervision group for four to five music therapists working with children with special needs in the Cambridge area.

In this chapter I shall reflect on receiving and giving supervision. Six of my supervisees have very kindly written about the experience of receiving supervision. Their stories make up the bulk of this chapter.

Receiving supervision

During the last 18 years I have had a number of different clinical supervisors from various professions, including psychiatric nurses, social workers, psychotherapists and clinical psychologists. Monthly supervision has been paid for by the NHS, as part of my music therapy post in child and family psychiatry. This has obviously been a great advantage, but it has meant that I have never had a music therapist as a clinical supervisor as there has not been another music therapist with experience in my field working for my employer.

When I first started having supervision, I remember worrying about whether my supervisor would make interpretations about my work that I would not agree with, or whether I would be asked difficult questions, or put on the spot. I felt it was important to impress my supervisor that I was a good clinician and only gradually gained the confidence to present or discuss those aspects of my work that I felt embarrassed about. As the years have gone by I have gained more confidence, and have found it easier to trust each new supervisor with aspects of my work that worry or upset me. I really value the opportunity to air my doubts, and my supervisors have always been encouraging and positive, making me feel good and excited about the work I was doing, or helping me to accept that some aspects of my work are very difficult and may not easily be resolved. Knowing I always had a supervision session to look forward to has meant that I have been able to put some clinical concerns aside to be reflected upon at a later stage.

In recent years, the issues I have taken to supervision often relate to my teaching, to my relationships with colleagues and management, or to my research and writing, rather than only to my clinical work. I appreciate the fact that my present clinical supervisor is not only an experienced clinician but also has management and teaching expertise.

Initially, I was worried about alluding to connections between my clinical work and my personal life in clinical supervision sessions. I felt that my home life and my professional life should be kept separate and I could not allow myself to talk about anything that was not directly connected to work. Many years of contact with skilled supervisors have taught me that the two worlds are not disconnected. Issues in my personal life that directly affect or are affected by my work can be usefully aired and explored, allowing me to reflect in constructive ways on how experiences and relationships at home and at work can enhance and inform one another.

I look forward to my clinical supervision sessions and feel they are a necessary part of my working life. During the sessions I feel looked after and valued but also challenged and stretched. I appreciate the time to think and reflect about all aspects of my work.

Giving individual supervision

Practical arrangements

Most of the music therapists I have supervised have come for an hour on a fortnightly or monthly basis. Some have a regular time every fortnight or month, others make arrangements for the next supervision from session to session. Usually supervision takes place at the Croft Unit for Child and Family Psychiatry where I have access to video equipment, but sometimes I have supervised at the university or at my home.

At present I am supervising four music therapists and I have been supervising roughly this number of people at any one time for the past ten years. The average length of time I have supervised people has been about three years.

Nearly all the music therapists I have supervised work with children or families. A few have worked with adults with learning difficulties and several have had a number of different jobs working with a wide range of client groups.

Some music therapists will pay for supervision sessions privately, others will be able to claim back some or all of the funds from their employer, and I provide supervision for one music therapist who works for my NHS trust, as part of my music therapy post.

The way I work as a clinical supervisor has developed and evolved through doing it rather than through learning a particular supervision technique or applying a specific theoretical approach.

General comments

Initially I explain that I am there to answer any work-related questions and that the topics covered in supervision will be determined by the supervisee. However, I always encourage music therapists to bring carefully chosen videotaped excerpts of sessions to supervision as often as possible as I strongly believe that examining videotapes of one's own work is one of the best ways of reflecting about the work and gaining new insights and skills. The learning takes place not only in supervision sessions themselves but also through viewing the videos, selecting excerpts and being clear what questions need to be asked in supervision.

Frequently, music therapists will find that when viewing videos of their own work it is not as 'bad' as they felt it was. This allows us to examine whether they are feeling anxious and perhaps therefore not aware that there are positive aspects to the work as well as difficult moments. Viewing videos also allows me to feed back what my musical responses might have been, or make suggestions for different approaches or alternative strategies. However, I also emphasise that there is hardly ever only one possible or correct course of action.

In Chapter 8, I wrote about the experience of having music therapy students on clinical placement. There are many similarities in my approach to supervising these students and supervising qualified music therapists. In both cases I feel it is important to build on existing strengths and emphasise positive aspects of the work. I also feel it is important to help music therapists to continue to be in touch with their own passion for music, as maintaining enthusiasm for music making is essential in order to remain creative and inspired during clinical improvisations.

Two music therapists that I have supervised individually have very kindly written moving reports about their experiences. I gave them some rough guidelines (see Appendix 10) but they have used very different styles, which I have not changed. I have worked with Philippa Derrington for five years, and during some of that time she also came to the supervision group that is described later in this chapter. She has been working on her MA and I have supervised this separately in addition to on-going monthly clinical supervision sessions. Emma Davies worked as my research assistant for three years and has been my music therapy colleague for six years. She has clinical supervision sessions with me every two or three weeks.

Philippa

Philippa writes: Clinical supervision with Amelia has helped me to clarify my thoughts and develop and shape my own approach to working as a music therapist whilst keeping me focused on the work and my therapeutic aims. Supervision is an intrinsic part of my clinical work, and while I find it important to think about specific cases, the process of discussing one case in detail impacts on my thinking and therefore on my work as a whole.

When I was first qualified I drew directly from Amelia's clinical ideas and felt supported by her experience and practical tools that worked well with children. For example, I was working at a primary school with a small group of children who all had varying needs, and I was finding it difficult to address the balance of working with each child in the group whilst engaging them all. Amelia's advice included thinking about ways of dividing up a session, as if into chunks, which each had a reason and purpose, and provided a sense of expectancy and fun. This method helped me to work in a clearer way and to think more imaginatively, such as adding movement and using other materials for a particular activity, or 'chunk'. This then allowed us all as a group to proceed therapeutically rather than chaotically.

Supervision has also been invaluable with issues that surround the clinical work. When I began working in secondary comprehensive schools I found Amelia's supervision to be, above all, encouraging. Her realistic and sensible approach to problems that naturally arise in staff groups helped me to cope with the commotion and challenges of setting up music therapy in this environment, and I felt positive about the work.

Supervision can offer a different perspective, rather like seeing work in three dimensions instead of one. For example, I took a piece of work with one teenager to supervision because I had a sense that we were getting stuck and there was little change. However, when I watched some of the work on video and began to notice interactions that Amelia was noticing, I recognised that there was more happening than I had felt or realised and became aware of ways in which to move the work forward.

Whilst I recognise the need to be flexible and student-centred in my work with teenagers, I incorporate structures which are a result of clear supervision and Amelia's consistent approach. I have found this method to be effective with these students. By establishing an overall structure, teenagers seem readier to express themselves in creative and improvised playing than if the structure was not in place. As much as teenagers may prefer to do things their own way, they are also used to following rules and school patterns and respond well to some direction.

Over time, supervision has become more about dialogue and discussion. I value Amelia's advice as an experienced music therapist but also recognise supervision as a sounding board for my own thoughts. So it is about the process of being supervised and reflecting on your own development as a therapist, as well as a channel for reflection, feedback and advice. It is also about sharing enthusiasm for music therapy.

Emma

Emma writes: I have had supervision with Amelia for the last five-and-a-half years. Throughout this time, my working life has gone through many challenging and exciting developments and I have worked with many different children and their families. Supervision has played, and I am sure will continue to play, a vital part of my development as a music therapist.

So what is Amelia's approach and how has it been so useful to me? Amelia works in a very open-minded way. She is not restricted to any set model of supervising, rather she listens and offers ideas that are relevant to each case or situation. She creates an environment in which I feel I can discuss anything, no matter how difficult. She often encourages me to show video extracts from my sessions which I find particularly helpful as she can provide objective thinking and ideas. Also she observes behaviours or responses that I do not always see, for example if I am working intensely with a family group. She has an infectious enthusiasm, not only for music and music therapy but also for life. She has an ability to get straight to the pertinent issues and can turn something that feels very difficult and uncontainable into something much more manageable.

When I first started supervision with Amelia, as a newly qualified therapist, I found showing videos of my work quite nerve-racking. I felt exposed and worried whether she would think I was any good. I suppose on a deeper level I felt rather like a child wanting to impress their teacher. However, as our working relationship continued and developed, I realised that it was through bringing up difficult issues and being prepared to admit when I find something challenging, that I was able to learn and move on as a therapist.

I would like to now discuss a case in which I found supervision incredibly helpful. A couple of years ago I worked with a ten-year-old boy who was diagnosed with severe psychosomatic symptoms. He was in an extreme state of anxiety when he was admitted to the unit where we both work. He was unable to walk, talk or even, at one point, eat. He crawled by dragging himself along the ground and sobbed or howled continuously. It was the first time I had ever seen anything like this and it was very difficult to watch. However, throughout his six months on the unit I saw him for both group and individual music therapy; the experience of which I will never forget. I talked a lot about this case with Amelia, openly discussing my own feelings as well as showing her video extracts to analyse.

Even though this was a very difficult case, Amelia always found something positive to draw from the sessions and made me realise that sometimes seemingly small acts hold huge significance, such as the act of this child crawling to the music room twice a week to see me. Through this case in particular, Amelia made me realise the importance not only of what kind of music therapist you are, but also what kind of person you are.

Previously I sometimes felt that there should be a *right* thing to say or do but I realised that this is not the case and you have to trust in your own approach, informed by experience and sensitivity. With Amelia's encouragement, I wrote a paper on this case and presented it at an international conference. Seeing her sitting on the front row of the audience, looking so enthusiastic, gave me so much confidence and helped me with my performance nerves. And perhaps a little bit of that 'child' in me was pleased that I could do something to impress her!

I work with children with a wide range of learning and physical disabilities as well as those with severe and complex psychiatric disorders. Most of my work involves working with children's families. Amelia has provided advice, support and insight in this area. She has been very adept at understanding the pace at which I should work, for example, offering a lot of time and space for children with severe disabilities.

With such a large caseload, it can be difficult to decide which case to bring to supervision. However, there is usually one that stands out and by dealing with some of the issues from one case, it can help with others.

As in any relationship, I have had to work at using supervision and I hope it will develop to reflect my own development and our work together. I would like to develop the psychodynamic thinking behind my work and do my own research, both of which I know Amelia will fully support. Sometimes supervision can feel a bit informal, perhaps because Amelia and I have worked together so intensely and have a friendship beyond our work. But then this is partly what makes me feel so supported and at ease in supervision, and what retains the enjoyment and fun of our work.

A supervision group

The supervision group was for music therapists employed by the Cambridge Instrumental Music Agency (CIMA), who were all working with children with special needs in special or mainstream schools in Cambridgeshire. Some of the music therapists worked for a few hours in a large number of different schools while others spent several days working in one school.

The group was set up in response to an increase in music therapists employed by CIMA. I no longer had the time available to supervise each of these music therapists on an individual basis, and we all felt that it would be useful to learn from each other's case presentations within a group setting.

The group took place once every six weeks, in the evening, and lasted for four years. Attendance varied from three to five as music therapists moved from one job to another, or went on extended study leave or maternity leave. For the first three years the group was run in the homes of the music therapists taking part in the group. At the end of each session the time and place of the next session would be decided. In the fourth year, as numbers increased the group moved to the music therapy room at the Croft children's unit. The length of each session varied from two to two-and-a-half hours, depending on how many people attended. We would break for drinks, biscuits and cakes.

For the first ten to fifteen minutes, as people arrived, we would chat informally and catch up with each other's news. I would then find out what everyone's needs were; which cases or groups were to be presented, what video excerpts were to be shown and any other issues that needed to be discussed. Most of the music therapists in the group presented cases every time we had a session, but occasionally music therapists would prefer to talk about a more general issue – regarding establishing music therapy within a new school, for example, or working with an overpowering support assistant.

The group ended after four years, for a combination of reasons. Some group members had been in the group for a long time and we all agreed that they would benefit from a change of clinical supervision arrangements. Other members were moving to different jobs or going on maternity leave. In addition, the CIMA team had by then become too large for all the music therapists to come to one supervision group. Some of the newcomers to CIMA wanted to see me for individual supervision rather than in a group.

I very much enjoyed running this group and learnt a tremendous amount from supervising a wide range of clinical work within a group setting. It is likely that I will run similar groups in the future as the need arises.

Four music therapists who took part in this group – Kathryn Nall, Elinor Everitt, Susan Greenhalgh and Jo Tomlinson – wrote about their experiences and the following are excerpts. I gave them some rough guidelines of what they might want to write about (see Appendix 11). Many thanks to the four of them for taking the time to write such honest and moving accounts. It is interesting to see that, although some impressions are similar, each individual wrote about slightly different aspects of the group.

Kathryn's perspective
There was almost a sense of celebration when we got together, a buzz of exchanges and never a shortage of either material to present or issues to discuss. Five therapists seemed to be a practical number for this group, but as with any group work it can feel frustrating to have to share the time. However, getting feedback, and having time to share with others made up for this. Once the group was set up it became apparent that the advantage of

such a group was that we all shared common problems and concerns. Most of us often worked in isolation within schools and had few opportunities to meet and discuss work with other therapists.

It could feel difficult in a group situation if time was running short and I had not managed to bring forward a problem I had wanted to share about a particularly difficult piece of work. However, Amelia usually managed to apportion time and enabled the group to feel sufficiently safe for people to share some of their most problematic pieces of work as well as those which had gone well.

There is inevitably some anxiety in presenting work to a group. "What will people think of me and my work if I show video clips of difficult moments?" It is very easy to edit these out and just show the positive parts of a session. As the group began to feel safe I came to realise that I did not always want to look at the "best" bits, in fact I gained most support and insight from being brave enough to look at the most difficult behaviour or emotions.

It seemed that for me, my recall of a music therapy session could be affected by a few minutes of difficulty. An example is a 12-year-old boy with severe autism. He had some language but most of this was echolalic and he had also developed a range of behaviours which all the staff were finding hard to cope with. In music therapy he would fling instruments to the ceiling with little or no warning, with no discrimination as to whether these might break or even hurt someone. What I had failed to remember were the parts of the session in which there had been sustained interaction. He had explored a reed horn carefully, pulled it apart and then at my suggestion began to very carefully repair it. We discussed how for these moments there was interaction and co-operation.

It was very helpful for me to have others comment and look at what may be happening and share ideas of how the work might move forward, when for me it had felt stuck. For myself I felt I needed to gauge how vulnerable I could allow myself to be and I believe this was something the other group members also had to grapple with. It seemed that the most helpful supervisions for me were those where I felt able to become vulnerable and I saw how this could then enable others to open up about their difficulties or feelings about the work. In addition, I was able to gain from looking at other people's work and hearing about their concerns.

From time to time feelings would well up, which might, for example, relate to how successful someone else seemed to be in dealing with a particular problem. Occasionally I felt envious: e.g. why does X always seem to have the most "musical" and able clients, what stunning improvisation, I could never do that…etc. Facilitated by our supervisor I was able to bring some of these thoughts out into the open, and often receive very positive comments about features of my own work. In sharing my vulnerabilities I have found a wealth of support for my own ideas and my own way of working, and my confidence has increased. I felt I needed this "secure place" where I could look at my "worst" work (as well as my best), without a fear of judgement or ridicule.

Working in isolation can make me feel vulnerable and defensive about my music therapy skills. Having a safe group within which to share both the good and the difficult work helped me to evaluate my work and to put my own skills and professional needs into perspective. Within the group I found an opportunity for peer support, and a sharing of mutual interests. I felt we all learnt an enormous amount from thinking about our work with others and being able to share our feelings and ideas for change.

Elinor's perspective
The group gave me the chance to meet up with my music therapy colleagues to share case studies or general difficulties and often provided me with much needed ideas.

I particularly found helpful the discussions about a child I was working with who had complex emotional and social needs resulting in behavioural difficulties. This boy was referred to me by his class teacher, who had seen his creative potential, and had wondered whether music therapy would provide a suitable outlet for him to explore various issues in his life.

The group helped me to focus on the positives of my work with him, such as the importance of providing him with a space to 'be', where he could be creative and feel good about himself. As the music therapy progressed we also discussed how as he could be a very controlling child I needed to lead and challenge him musically, as well as following his music and ideas, making it clear that we took turns to choose different aspects of the session.

The group provided me with a chance to talk about how I felt with regard to working with this difficult child. Often his stories were violent or about war, with loud perseverative drumming frequently being a feature. Thinking about the different ways in which these stories were or could be resolved was helpful. It was also suggested that I should watch out for and develop his more playful side in our music and interactions.

A lot of the services and agencies found working with this child challenging and seemed to focus on the more negative side of his character. I felt
that his music therapy was a very positive part of his life, so the group
discussed how important it was that I put this across to the other services
involved in working with him.

Towards the end of my work with him, his school attendance became
less predictable and there were uncertainties with regard to his future school
arrangements. I needed to think about how I might finish this piece of work
and how it was likely to be an unsatisfactory conclusion. I therefore changed
the words of our 'goodbye' song to 'I hope to see you next week', acknowledging that neither of us could be certain of what might happen in the
coming week with regards his behaviour, school attendance and which
school he might be attending the following academic year.

Susan's perspective

The group was fun, interesting, inspiring and exciting. The atmosphere was
relaxed, non-threatening and encouraging. It was something I looked
forward to.

The material I brought to the group varied. Often it might have been a
case that I was finding overwhelmingly challenging. I remember one case
when I was working with a young teenage twin. Both of the boys were
attending the same school, and the relationship between them evoked strong
feelings of envy and jealousy. Both boys had an extremely sad and emotionally difficult background from an early age. The twin, John, that I was
working with used the music therapy space in a variety of ways. On some
occasions, John would just sit and be unable to play anything either on his
own or with me. John always looked sad. On other occasions, John would
portray his amazing musicality, and share a ten-minute improvisation often
on the glockenspiel (sharing it with me or me playing the piano). John's
sadness was overwhelming. His dismissive approach following his exciting
musical playing (usually by throwing the beaters across the room) was
something I found disturbing. His self-esteem was low, he was unable to
accept anything good he had done, either in class or in the music therapy
room. In the group we began to look at the implications of being a twin.
John was a boy who was always in more trouble at home than his twin. He
would therefore be denied treats as a result of his behaviour. Both the school
staff and I felt that this, coupled with his abusive childhood, was a primary

cause of his depression. This child was the most severely depressed that I had worked with, both then and now.

I was looking for answers and wanted a resolution in order to help him manage his sadness. This child had a great sense of loss. As a child he was left alone with his twin brother, for many hours, locked up in a room without food. I was craving to give him a happy, positive experience. During the group discussion about John, the whole issue of how to move the therapy forward for him became clearer.

Playing music together in the individual sessions was giving him a positive experience, but it was going to take a long time for him to take on board that he is good at doing this, and that he is special. Therefore repetition was necessary over a period of time, to improve his self-esteem. For him to have a special place without his brother was important. He needed a safe, one-to-one setting where he knew that I was setting aside time for him alone, to explore aspects of himself. In this setting, I was eventually able to help him to articulate his painful thoughts verbally alongside the positive musical experiences. Discussing John in supervision has remained with me, and I am able to recall this case and how I was influenced by the group whenever I work with severely depressed adolescents and children.

In my opinion bringing material to a supervision group has some benefits that are not found in individual supervision. For example in a group of several therapists, there is going to be a larger range of musical material and ideas and I found it healthy to experience a diversity of approaches. However, I felt that working in a group did take a bit of practice. For the initial months of the group I did often feel concerned about how people would react to my work. However, the more I did present, the less I worried. Difficulties were shared. People were encouraging and gave constructive criticism.

I thought the group had a good balance between formal and informal. There was always a relaxed atmosphere, and one where a sense of humour was paramount. For me, this was important, as I think humour can enable us to learn and remember. The group was an extremely happy experience for me.

Jo's perspective

Initially I found that I brought pieces of work to the supervision group that I felt confident about presenting, but as the group evolved I became more secure about bringing work that I was anxious about or 'stuck' with. I found the group to be extremely supportive and fascinating to be a part of. The group supervision seemed to pass very quickly and we would often go on discussing music therapy until late into the evening. Amelia's advice was always extremely useful and instructive and it was also helpful to get feed-back and insight from discussion with other group members. It was reassuring to know that other members of the group were working with clients with similar problems in a school context, and the challenges that this presented in music therapy sessions.

I felt a transition occurred for me when I was appointed Head of Music Therapy for CIMA. I initially had concerns that my new role might affect the discussion that took place within the group, as I suddenly had 'performance management' responsibilities for the team. I was not sure how this would impact on therapists' openness about discussing work that appeared problematic. I talked to Amelia about this and then we had a discussion during a supervision group about the issue. We concluded that it should not create difficulties in relation to supervision of the work as my role as performance manager was in a supportive rather than a judgemental capacity. The positive outcome would be that I would keep in touch with music therapy that was evolving in school settings around the county.

In the supervision group I discussed my music therapy work with a child called Peter. Peter was nine years old and had a diagnosis of autism. Peter attended the special needs school at which I work for three days a week.

During the period of time that I worked with Peter some behavioural patterns emerged which corresponded with Peter's relationships with other people at the school. Peter was extremely controlling within sessions and avoided any type of shared interactive exchange. He moved frenetically around the music therapy room, constantly avoiding contact with me and carrying out purely mechanical exploration of the musical instruments. Peter was very rejecting of both my musical and non-musical intervention and this made the sessions feel extremely challenging.

Peter was not overly responsive to music but could become focused on specific songs that his mother had recommended to me. These were mostly songs that he had listened to within the context of television programmes. This type of material sometimes provided a 'way in' to more direct communication with him.

I took this piece of work for supervision because I was finding it difficult to establish ways of engaging with Peter within sessions. I felt rejected by him, both musically and personally, and was experiencing similar feelings to the other adults at the school who worked with Peter. I was additionally conscious of Peter getting into negative behaviour patterns with other people and was keen to avoid any confrontational exchanges within the music therapy setting.

I discussed this case in two group supervision sessions over the period of time that I was working with Peter. Within supervision I was able to reflect on my relationship with Peter and the dynamics of our communication. I was also able to consider practical strategies for dealing with his avoidance of me.

Analysing the dynamics of my relationship with Peter and transference/countertransference issues was essential for me in retaining a constructive attitude towards music therapy with him. Peter made me feel as if there was an impenetrable barrier between us in terms of communication. This could have led to frustration and irritation permeating our relationship. I felt that my role as therapist was to support, develop communication channels, provide a medium for self-expression, and facilitate positive interaction. Peter's resistance to my communicative exchanges made me feel powerless and enabled him to retain a sense of control. Through discussing this dynamic within supervision I was able to focus on my relationship with Peter in a more constructive way. I was able to analyse the feelings that Peter naturally provoked within me, consider the possible detrimental impact of these feelings on our relationship, and consequently establish alternative responses to him. Through processing these feelings within a contained space I was able to maintain clear boundaries and consider ways of working with Peter which would enhance the therapeutic potential of sessions. It was also helpful to consider that Peter might at times be automatically rejecting me because of his inability to make communicative connections or cope with any sense of togetherness.

The impact of supervision on this case study was therefore to help me understand the dynamics which were evolving between Peter and myself. This enabled me to view the relationship from a new perspective and facilitated my capacity to work constructively alongside Peter's social and communicative difficulties. Analysing the reasons for his behaviour and considering ways of increasing his levels of security in sessions also enabled Peter to engage with me with greater flexibility and trust.

On a more practical level, we discussed strategies for coping with Peter's avoidance of me. We discussed Peter's desire to control any interaction that occurred within sessions. This meant that I constantly felt that I was 'chasing' Peter to encourage him to engage in some way with me. Amelia suggested two different strategies with which to respond to this.

One strategy was for me to remain static and focus in on something myself to see if Peter would become curious about my activity; for example, studying the strings of the guitar and slowly plucking them. The other response was to move around the room in a faster or more unusual way than Peter to see if we could alter the balance of this interchange. We discussed the element of surprise and breaking out of established patterns in sessions.

Both of these strategies worked to a degree and promoted a change in our relationship. Peter seemed to begin to perceive me as less intrusive and consequently diminished his avoidance of me. Although our direct communication within sessions was minimal, the interaction we did have had a greater feeling of connectedness. Overall there was less resistance and indirect aggression.

Supervision, therefore, enabled me to view my music therapy work with Peter with greater clarity and insight. It helped me to step back psychologically from my relationship with him and consider ways in which to respond to him that would be constructive in relation to the therapeutic process. It also provided me with insight into my own feelings about the work and enabled me to consider the potential impact of this on my relationship with Peter. Essentially, supervision created a space for reflection, discussion and analysis, leaving me feeling simultaneously challenged and supported in my role as music therapist.

Reflections on what supervisees have written

First, it was wonderful for me to read that the people I had supervised felt so positive about supervision, thought that the sessions had been useful and had learnt from the experience.

There were a few aspects of supervision that were mentioned by nearly all the music therapists. One was that at first they were nervous about showing video excerpts of their music therapy sessions. They started by showing excerpts where they felt that they were working very well and only gradually plucked up the courage to show excerpts where they felt they were not working so successfully. However, once they did have the confidence to show their 'worst' work they found this a very supportive and helpful process.

Another aspect of supervision that was frequently mentioned was how the music therapists were helped to focus on their own strengths and the parts of the sessions that were working well rather than being overwhelmed by difficult moments, or their own feelings of inadequacy.

The process of gathering together impressions from six music therapists I have supervised, and writing this chapter, has enabled me to learn more about the way I supervise. In future, for example, I will be more aware of music therapists' initial fears and continue to encourage them to focus on all aspects of their sessions rather than only on the problems they perceive.

Conclusion

As earlier chapters in this book and as Oldfield (2006) have shown, I very much enjoy and am fascinated by both my clinical work and teaching others about music therapy. It is, therefore, not surprising that talking about my work (receiving supervision) and hearing about other music therapists' work (giving supervision) is equally enjoyable and interesting.

In my own supervision I am not only supported and encouraged, but gain a sense of perspective and can reflect, and gain new insights. When giving supervision I see a wide range of clinical work and many different music therapy approaches, styles and techniques. I attempt to support, reflect and make suggestions and at the same time new ideas about clinical music therapy will constantly be emerging.

Conclusion

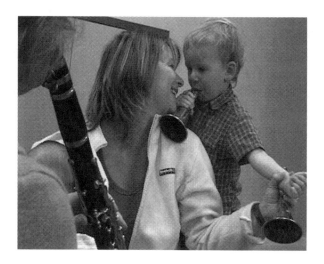

In this book, I have used the term 'interactive music therapy' to describe the way I work as a music therapist at the Croft Unit for Child and Family Psychiatry. This approach was first defined in a companion book (Oldfield 2006) which is about my work at a Child Development Centre. In it I outlined a series of points that were central to my work with parents and pre-school children. These points were different depending on whether the children were on the autistic spectrum, had severe physical and mental learning difficulties or had identified difficulties but no clear diagnosis. However, with all three client groups it was clear that the focus was primarily on the interactive processes between the therapist and the child, between the child and the parent and between the therapist and the parent.

In the introductory chapter of the present book I make several general points about my music therapy approach in child and family psychiatry. These are:

- Musical interactions are at the centre of my work. It is through the non-verbal improvised musical exchanges that I can engage and capture children's and parents' interest and attention.

- The focus is not only on the relationship between myself and the child but also on the relationship between the child and the parent and between the parent and myself. The quality of these relationships is important, even when my work is short-term and consists of only one or two sessions.

- The positive aspect of the music therapy experience is often of paramount importance.

- Therapeutic teaching may play a part in my work.

- My work and approach has to be flexible and I have to respond to the needs of children and families as they arise, sometimes adjusting my timetable on the day I arrive.

- The value of my work at the Croft is dependent on working closely with the psychiatric team, liaising and feeding back on a daily and weekly basis.

In Chapters 2, 3, 4 and 5, I describe different types of music therapy interventions at the Croft. Additional characteristics of my music therapy approach emerge in each of these specific areas. For example, in my Music Therapy Diagnostic Assessments (Chapter 2) my focus is particularly on observing children's strengths and weaknesses in non-verbal interactions. In the group (Chapter 3), issues of control are often at the centre of my work, and in the work with families (Chapter 5), I may be particularly interested in how parents perceive their children's strengths and weaknesses.

In each of the different clinical areas, I refer to other music therapists' approaches and ways of working and examine differences and similarities in styles of work. Although there are aspects of my work which overlap with that of other music therapists, the points I draw out of my clinical work seem to characterise and be typical of my 'interactive music therapy' approach.

The first five chapters have 22 vignettes and case studies. This shows that my clinical work is (and continues to be) at the root of all my thinking. However, the research described in Chapters 6 and 7 has clarified and confirmed my thoughts about my clinical practice. In Chapter 6, I have looked at the common points in my different research investigations and made some suggestions that may be helpful to music therapists who are considering embarking on research. In addition to helping me to define and clarify my approach, I have found the process of research exciting and stimulating. I think that the research I have undertaken has helped me to become a better clinician.

The final two chapters (Chapters 8 and 9) reflect on my experience of teaching music therapy and of music therapy supervision. Nearly all music therapists will be involved in running some workshops and teaching sessions in the places where they work. I therefore thought it might be useful to describe a music therapy workshop format in some detail. I have found that talking and teaching about music therapy is another way to clarify my own thoughts about music therapy processes, especially when I am questioned and challenged by the people I am teaching.

I have also really enjoyed and learnt from teaching music therapy students and have described various aspects of my role in training music therapists in Chapter 8. Preparing lectures, running workshops and answering searching questions asked by music therapy students have helped me to learn to describe my work clearly and understand the reasons behind the choices and decisions I take.

Writing my final Chapter 9 on supervision has been a very rewarding experience because of the reports written by six of my supervisees. Seeing work carried out by other music therapists has not only been interesting and enjoyable but has been another factor that has helped me to define my own approach.

I am aware that there is literature written by music therapists about teaching and supervision that I have not referred to in this book. Unlike the earlier chapters where I have studied the literature and carried out research to put my work into context, Chapters 8 and 9 are purely descriptive and reflective. I hope to read more, and possibly set up some research in this area in future.

In some ways writing down thoughts about my work is a little like trying to capture a moment within a music therapy improvisation. As soon as it is described, the moment has passed and is no longer quite the same. The context has changed, other factors need to be taken into consideration. I will have also slightly changed and my perspective will be a little different. My ideas about my work are constantly changing and developing. After 25 years, I am still challenged and I still learn from the families I treat, from the workshops I run and from the music therapists I supervise. It is a fascinating experience.

I hope that the 'moment' that this book represents contains information that will be useful to others interested in music therapy.

Blank sheet (usually on distinctive pink paper) used for recording on-going music therapy notes in the Croft nursing folder

Music Therapy Notes

Name: General Croft Aims:

Date: **Group session** **Individual session** **Family session** (select one)	
Date: **Group session** **Individual session** **Family session** (select one)	
Date: **Group session** **Individual session** **Family session** (select one)	
Date: **Group session** **Individual session** **Family session** (select one)	
Date: **Group session** **Individual session** **Family session** (select one)	

Summary describing Damien's music therapy session on 16 November 1999*

Music Therapy Notes

Name: Damien Smith   **General Croft Aims:** To assess for ADD (attention deficit disorder) and ASD autistic spectrum disorder)

Date: 9.11.1999 **Individual session**	Damien seemed content to come with me when I collected him from the classroom. He was quietly compliant, conforming with my requests but not initiating anything verbally. In our improvised drum and piano exchange he appeared to become more animated, at times playing quite loudly and forcefully. He was able to listen to and follow my musical suggestions and, gradually, as his confidence increased, initiated a few of his own rhythmic phrases. He concentrated well. His speech intonation was a little unusual. Signed: A. Oldfield, music therapist
Date: 10.11.1999 **Group session**	Damien was a quiet member of the group, taking part in all suggested musical interactions and games, but not speaking up or initiating any ideas of his own either verbally or non-verbally. He was happy to lead the group and acknowledged praise from his peers, but in a 'matter of fact' way without showing emotion. He was not distractible and unaware of other peers' efforts to draw him into rebellious behaviours. At one point he told another peer to stop being 'a naughty boy'. Signed: A. Oldfield, music therapist

Date: 16.11.1999 **Individual session**	Damien obviously enjoyed playing the instruments and demonstrated a good sense of pitch and phrasing, singing musically and in tune. Although quiet at first, he soon became quite animated, particularly in our improvised song story. He told a story about a naughty boy who smashed plates and was locked in his bedroom. He was very spontaneous and made most of the suggestions in the story; however he was also able to listen to and incorporate my contributions. I would like to show a video of the session to the team as I was concerned about his excitement about imaginary violence and chaos. Signed: A. Oldfield, music therapist

*   Notes from previous sessions are also included on the form. The notes on 16 November relate to the vignette in Chapter 1. These notes would usually be written by hand.

Appendix 3

Summary describing Nancy, Claude and Phoebe's music therapy session

Music Therapy Notes

Name: Nancy, Claude and Phoebe Jones

General Croft Aims: Parenting assessment; increasing Nancy's confidence

Date: 10.11.1999 **Family session**	Nancy was warm and caring with both her children and they clearly showed that they were used to this caring approach from their mother by snuggling up to her or seeking reassurance from her when anything new or unusual was presented. Nancy was shy about playing at first but allowed herself to be drawn into playing the reed horns by Claude. In their exchange, Claude played the horn in his mother's ear and she became very playful, making faces, pretending to back away, and laughing with Claude. After the session Nancy said that she enjoyed playing the instruments with the children although she hadn't expected to. We agreed to continue with weekly sessions that we would video. Signed: A. Oldfield, music therapist

Damien's music therapy report

Music Therapy Report

Name: Damien Smith

Date: 20.12.1999

Damien took part in two music therapy assessment sessions and four group music therapy sessions during his admission at the Croft.

Individual sessions

Damien enjoyed playing the instruments and singing during his individual sessions. He was not self-conscious or worried about how well he would play. He showed a good sense of pitch, rhythm and phrasing. At first he was quite quiet, but then he gradually become more involved with the instruments and played quite loudly and spontaneously. In our improvisations, he was able to follow my musical suggestions as well as initiate his own.

When making up a song-story in his second session, Damien became very involved and excited, shouting suggestions for the story and waiting for me to echo these back to him with musical accompaniment before shouting the next suggestion. The story was about a naughty boy who smashed plates and was punished by both his mother and his father. He was quite repetitive in this story, suggesting again and again that more plates were smashed, but was able to move on and bring the story to a close when I prompted him. His excitement about the violence and deviance in this made-up story was very different from his usual quiet and compliant manner. He also shouted and laughed loudly while telling the story, whereas at other times he spoke in a quiet voice with little changes of intonation.

He never had any difficulties concentrating and was not distractible.

Group sessions

Damien took part quietly in group sessions, although in the later groups he would sometimes play instruments quite loudly during group playing. He understood instructions and joined in with all the musical games. He was quite watchful and appeared to use non-verbal cues more easily than spoken language. He was happy to play a solo on his own or conduct his peers, but did this in a slightly 'bland' way, not showing a great sense of achievement or particular pleasure when he was praised by adults or peers. He did not react to peers' enticements to be deviant or naughty, simply ignoring their cues. On several occasions he told other children that they were being naughty and appeared to expect adults to react, but again this did not appear to be in order to cause problems for other children but rather as a statement of fact.

Recommendations

Damien enjoys playing the musical instruments and finds it easy to play freely and spontaneously. In song-stories particularly, he becomes very involved and excited. This level of involvement and expression was not observed in any other setting during his stay at the Croft. If individual music therapy sessions were available (either in Damien's school or in a clinic that he could access), I would recommend that Damien has further individual music therapy sessions in order to have a chance to express himself through his playing and through imaginary song-stories. It is possible that some of the violent outbursts that have been reported at home would decrease if Damien had this opportunity to express his feelings in a constructive way.

Signed: A. Oldfield, music therapist

Nancy, Claude and Phoebe's music therapy report

Music Therapy Report

Names: The Jones family, Nancy (mother), Claude (2) and Phoebe (11 weeks)

Date: 12.1.2000

Nancy, Claude and Phoebe took part in four family music therapy sessions during their attendance at the Croft.

Nancy was initially shy about coming to music therapy sessions because she felt that she was not particularly good at music. However, when Claude started playing the reed horns she became drawn into the musical exchange with him and was able to have fun and laugh with him. At first Claude was shy about playing the drums but by the third session he started to really enjoy playing both the drum and the cymbal, particularly when I followed his playing on the piano and his mother accompanied him on the tambourine. He enjoyed conducting us from the drums, grinning delightedly when we stopped as soon as he stopped. After this session Nancy told me that the session had gone really quickly because they were all really 'into' the music. She said that, at the weekend, she had tried dancing with Claude to a piece of music they heard on the radio – and they had both ended up in fits of giggles. She was more animated than I had seen her previously and her mood generally lifted as the weeks progressed.

During the sessions, baby Phoebe was very aware of the music going on around her and watched intently to where the sounds were coming from. She smiled often and only seldom was grizzly. Nancy was very good at holding her and attending to her while at the same time playing with Claude.

When I observed some video excerpts of our sessions with Nancy, she was embarrassed at first, saying she was sure she would look awful. When I pointed out how good she was at engaging Claude while at the same time looking after Phoebe she seemed surprised, but pleased, as though she was only just beginning to be able to recognise that she was being a good mother. At the end of her Croft admission, Nancy was pleased to take home a videotape of excerpts of family music therapy sessions. I also gave Nancy a list of musical games and songs she could use at home. I hope she continues to have fun through music with both her children.

Signed: A. Oldfield, music therapist

Croft group 'Hello' song

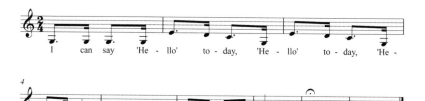

Full MTDA scoring sheets

Score in the following way:

0 = None of this behaviour was noticed

1 = Some of this behaviour was noticed

2 = A lot of this behaviour was noticed

NB: Only score if you are certain you noticed some of the behaviour. If in any doubt, do not score.

Autistic spectrum disorder categories

(a) Child's playing seems to be independent of therapist's playing. Therapist has to work hard to 'remain' with child, and child often seems to be doing his/her own thing.   Score …

(b) Child is not facially or physically engaged in playing process, or unusual eye-contact (too little or too much).   Score …

(c) Child does not make *any* spontaneous suggestions (musical or verbal) with communicative intent; or story is excessively simple, showing inability to be creative or imaginative (this should not be caused by a general learning disability, but appear untypical of the child's overall ability).   Score …

(d) Child is unusually interested in structure of instruments; lines instruments or beaters up; 'twiddles' with beaters or shakers; uses beaters in unexpected ways e.g. puts them in holes, sticks them on head…   Score …

(e) Child becomes self-absorbed and difficult to distract from certain instruments such as the wind chimes or the ocean drum (not boredom or distractability but a more isolated, engrossed type of playing, with possible repetitive playing).   Score …

(f) Child's tone of voice/intonation has an unusual or
repetitive quality.   Score ...

(g) Child is unable or unwilling to make up a story where we
both contribute to the storyline. Child may be unwilling
to make up a new story rather than telling a well-known
story, or child may refuse to allow the therapist to
contribute in any way.   Score ....

(h) Child develops obsessive/repetitive types of playing or
obsessive repetitive patterns in story.   Score ....

(i) Child is unable to have more than one immediate copying
response. The exchanges do not develop into a dialogue.
                                                               Score ....

(j) Child is unable to have any playful or humorous exchange
with the therapist.   Score ....

(k) Child wants entire session to be on his/her terms and
cannot accept any ideas or suggestions from the therapist
(not in a calculated manipulative way but rather in an
'own world' way).   Score ....

(l) Child does not show a response to therapist's singing. No
embarrassment or smile or communicative response. Do
not score if child is choosing to reject or ignore the
therapist and showing a negative response.   Score ....

                                                              Total ....

Attention deficit disorder

(m) Child has difficulties remaining engaged in any one   Score ...
activity for more than a few minutes.

(n) Child is very distractible and fiddles with beaters or
knobs on percussion instruments; child has difficulty
remaining in one place; child fidgets.   Score ...

                                                              Total ...

Emotional difficulties

(o) Child is very anxious, or finds it difficult making own choices; child seems to lack a sense of self.   Score ...

(p) Child has difficulties moving from one activity to another; child has difficulties coming to the session or leaving the session.   Score ...

(q) Child seems to need to be in control of session and therapist in a 'powerful' way rather than in order to be reassured about the session.   Score ...

(r) Child is defiant and seems to want to draw therapist into a conflict.   Score ...

(s) Child is impulsive and unpredictable.   Score ...

Total ...

Language or learning disabilities

(t) Child is difficult to understand; has pronunciation difficulties; speaks in an ungrammatical way (more so than age of child would lead you to expect).   Score ...

(u) Child speaks very little or not at all; or child seems very anxious about speaking. Do not score when therapist feels child is making a point of not speaking but only if it is felt that child has real difficulties in this area.   Score ...

(v) Child has difficulties understanding the therapist.   Score ...

(w) Child is clumsy or awkward/uncoordinated.   Score ...

Total ...

Cut-off points:

Autism: 10

Autistic spectrum: 6

Attention deficit disorder: 3

Emotional/difficulties: 4

Language/learning difficulties: 4

MTDA and ADOS testers' questionnaire (to be filled in straight after test)

Name of child:

Name of tester:

Date:

1. **Was test an effective tool?**
   Answer this question for each activity presented to child.
   Score in the following way: (a) very effective; (b) effective; (c) not very informative; (d) useless.

   Activity 1:

   Title ....

   Score ....

   Activity 2:

   Title ....

   Score ....

   Activity 3:

   Title ....

   Score ....

   Activity 4:

   Title ....

   Score ....

Activity 5:

Title ....

Score ....

Activity 6:

Title ....

Score ....

Activity 7:

Title ....

Score ....

Activity 8:

Title ....

Score ....

Activity 9:

Title ....

Score ....

Activity 10:

Title ....

Score ....

Activity 11:

Title ....

Score ....

Activity 12:

Title ....

Score ....

2. Did person carrying out test feel that they administered the test well?
(answer Yes or No and comment)

Yes ☐ No ☐

Comments:

3. What were the limitations of the test?
(immediate reactions)

Comments:

4. Particular immediate impressions of child – e.g. what stood out?

Comments:

5. Reactions of research assistant regarding whether child behaved in an expected or unexpected way during the session
(only relevant to Music Therapy Diagnostic Assessments)

Circle one:

Expected behaviour   Slightly unexpected   Very unexpected
                            behaviour   behaviour

Comments:

Guidelines for structured interviews with the children

This interview aims to give us information about:

- How the children perceive the MT diagnostic procedure and the ADOS.
- Whether the tests interest and engage the children.
- How children experience being with another adult; reciprocity; ability to empathise.
- We may find that some of the questions asked in this structured interview should be incorporated into the MT diagnostic procedure and/or the ADOS.

Motivation/interest

Choose the strand of the question that relates to the appropriate assessment (i.e. music therapy or ADOS).

- What did you like best, and what was your worst thing?
- Have you ever done any of these games (played any instruments or done any singing) before?

Experience of being with another adult

- Was it like other games you've played before with your family, or a friend; like playing instruments or singing at school; with a teacher; with a friend?
- Did you like taking turns?
- Did you like choosing, or did you prefer Jo or Amelia choosing?
- Was it fun being with Jo/Amelia?
- Did you like it better when you were playing alone?

Self-esteem/confidence

- You're quite good at doing puzzles; building towers; playing the drum. Is singing fun?
- It's a good feeling being good at things. Do you do these things at home/school with family/friends?
- Explore an obvious area of difficulty in a positive way. For example: It was hard thinking of ideas for the story, but you had a good idea at the end. Sometimes it takes time to think of things. I'm shy about singing too, but I like singing in the bath.

Perception of other person's feelings:

- What did you think Jo/Amelia liked best?
- Did they seem to enjoy themselves?
- Perhaps you both had fun together.

Guidelines for writing about individual supervision

Individual supervision with Amelia

Some questions that might be useful when thinking about supervision – only use if helpful, don't feel these questions have to be answered. Anything you write will be very much appreciated, whether it's a couple of paragraphs or several pages. THANK YOU!

- Describe one or two cases or pieces of work you brought to supervision. Why did you bring the material, was it helpful, what did you learn from Amelia, and/or from the process of discussing the case?
- How do you decide what material to bring to supervision?
- Have you felt different about your work as time has gone on? How?
- Has the way you felt about supervision or being in supervision changed? How?
- Is the supervision too formal/informal?
- Do you wish there were things you had discussed but didn't get around to after supervision had finished?
- Do you feel listened to?
- Are there things you particularly like about the supervision, things that you don't like, things you would like to change, add, develop?

Guidelines for writing about group supervision

Group clinical supervision run by Amelia for CIMA music therapists between 2000 and 2004

Some questions that might be useful when thinking back to the group – only use if helpful, don't feel these questions have to be answered. Anything you write will be very much appreciated, whether it's a couple of paragraphs or several pages. THANK YOU!

- Describe one or two cases or pieces of work you brought to the group. Why did you bring the material, was it helpful, what did you learn from Amelia, from the other group members, from the process of presenting the case?
- How did you decide what material to bring to supervision?
- Did you feel different about your work as time went on? How?
- Did the way you felt about the group or being in the group change? How?
- Why was it useful presenting material in a group rather than individually?
- Was the group too formal/informal?
- Did you feel listened to, or overwhelmed and/or frustrated?
- Did you feel you had a voice in the group?
- Did it change the group for you when it was run at the Croft rather than in different group member's homes? Advantages/disadvantages of this?
- When we stopped the group, did this seem to be at the right time? Was the ending OK?
- Are there things you particularly liked about the group, things that you didn't like, things you would have liked to change, add, develop?

References

Abidin, R. (1995) *Parenting Stress Index*. Professional manual for Psychological Assessment Resources Inc., USA.

Aldridge, D. (1996) *Music Therapy Research and Practice in Medicine: From Out of the Silence*. London: Jessica Kingsley Publishers.

Alvin, J. (1966) *Music Therapy*. London: John Clare Books.

Ansdell, A. and Pavlicevic, M. (2001) *Beginning Research in the Arts Therapies*. London: Jessica Kingsley Publishers.

APMT (1997) Music therapy leaflet, published by the Association of Professional Music Therapists.

Baron-Cohen, S. and Bolton, P. (1993) *Autism: the Facts*. Oxford: Oxford Medical.

Bean, J. and Oldfield, A. (2001) *Pied Piper: Musical Activities to Develop Basic Skills*. London: Jessica Kingsley Publishers.

Boxhill, E.H. (1985) *Music Therapy for the Developmentally Disabled*. Rockville, MD: Aspen Publications.

Bruscia, K. (1987) *Improvisation Models of Music Therapy*. Springfield, IL: Charles C. Thomas.

Bruscia, K. (1995) 'Differences between Quantitative and Qualitative Research Paradigms: Implications for Music Therapy.' In B. Wheeler (ed) *Music Therapy Research: Quantitative and Qualitative Perspectives*. Phoenixville, PA: Barcelona Publishers, 65–76.

Bunt, L. (2002) 'Suzanna's Story.' In L. Bunt and S. Hoskyns (eds) *The Handbook of Music Therapy*. East Sussex: Brunner–Routledge, 73–83.

Bunt, L. and Hoskyns, S. (eds) (2002) *The Handbook of Music Therapy*. East Sussex: Brunner-Routledge.

Bunt, L. and Pavlicevic, M. (2001) 'Music and Emotion: Perspectives from Music Therapy.' In N. Juslin and J. Sloboda (eds) *Music and Emotion, Theory and Research*. Oxford: Oxford University Press, 181–201.

Bunt, L., Pike, D. and Wren, V. (1987) 'Music Therapy in a General Hospital's Psychiatric Unit: A Pilot Evaluation of an Eight Week Programme.' *Journal of British Music Therapy 1*, 2, 22–27.

Carr, A. (1999) *The Handbook of Child and Adolescent Psychology, a Contextual Approach*. Hove and New York: Brunner-Routledge.

Carter, E. and Oldfield, A. (2002) 'A Music Therapy Group to assist Clinical Diagnoses in Child and Family Psychiatry.' In A. Davies and E. Richards (eds) *Group Work in Music Therapy*. London: Jessica Kingsley Publishers.

Dilavore, P., Rutter, M. and Lord, C. (1995) 'The Prelinguistic Autistic Diagnostic Schedule.' *Journal of Autism and Developmental Disorders 25*, 4, 355–79.

Dunachie, S. (1995) 'Perspectives on a Developmental Model of Music Therapy with Mentally Handicapped Adults.' In T. Wigram, B. Saperston and R. West (eds) *The Art and Science of Music Therapy: A Handbook*. Chur, Switzerland: Harwood Academic Publishers, 288–95.

Edwards, J. (1999a) 'Considering the Paradigmatic Frame: Social Science Research Approaches Relevant to Research in Music Therapy.' *The Arts in Psychotherapy, 26*, 2, 73–80.

Edwards, J. (1999b) 'Music Therapy with Children Hospitalised for Severe Injury or Illness.' *British Journal of Music Therapy, 13*, 1, 21–7.

Edwards, J. (2002) 'Using the Evidence Based Medicine Framework to Support Music Therapy Posts in Healthcare Settings.' *British Journal of Music Therapy 16*, 1, 29–34.

Ford, H. (1994) 'Parents Project.' *Young Minds Newsletter, 17.*

Freemann, B., Ritvo, E. and Schroth, P. (1984) 'Behaviour Assessment of the Syndrome of Autism: Behaviour Observation System.' *Journal of American Academy of Child Psychiatry, 23*, 588–94.

Froehlich, M.A. (1984) 'A Comparison of the Effect of Music Therapy and Medical Play Therapy on the Verbalisation Behaviour of Pediatric Patients.' *Journal of Music Therapy 21*, 1, 2–15.

Gfeller, K. (1995) 'The Status of Music Therapy Research.' In B. Wheeler (ed) *Music Therapy Research: Quantitative and Qualitative Perspectives.* Phoenixville, PA: Barcelona Publishers, 29–63.

Grant, R. (1995) 'Music Therapy Assessment for Developmentally Disabled Clients.' In T. Wigram, B. Saperston and R. West (eds) *The Art and Science of Music Therapy: A Handbook.* Chur, Switzerland: Harwood Academic Publishers, 273–87.

Griessmeier, B. (1994) *Musiktherapie mit Krebstkranken Kindern.* Stuttgart: Bärenreiter Verlag.

Hibben, J. (1991) 'Group Music Therapy with a Classroom of 6–8 year old Hyperactive Learning Disabled Children.' In K. Bruscia (ed) *Case Studies in Music Therapy.* Phoenixville, PA: Barcelona Publishers.

Howlin, P. (2003) 'The Evidence Base for Therapeutic Interventions for Autism.' Unpublished paper given on 3 November 2003 at the one-day conference 'Autism and Asperger's Syndrome' held at the Royal Society of Medicine Centre in London, organised by the Royal Society for Medicine.

Howlin, P. and Rutter, M. (1989) *Treatment of Autistic Children.* Chichester: John Wiley.

Isenberg-Grezda, I. (1988) 'Music Therapy Assessment: A Reflection of Professional Identity.' *Music Therapy 25*, 3, 156–69.

Lenz, G. (1996) 'Music Therapy and "Early Interactional Disorders": Example of the Cry Babies.' Unpublished paper presented at the 8th World Congress of Music Therapy, 'Sound and Psyche', Hamburg, Germany.

Levinge, A. (1993) 'The Nursing Couple.' Unpublished paper presented at the 7th World Congress of Music Therapy, Vitoria, Spain.

Levinge, A. (2000) 'Applying Winnicottian Theory in Music Therapy Research.' Unpublished paper presented at the 2nd Music Therapy Research Convivium, organised by the British Society for Music Therapy and City University, London, October.

Loewy, L.V. (1999) 'Medical Music Therapy Assessment.' In B. Wilson and E. York (co-chairs) *Proceedings of the Institute of Music Therapy Assessment.* World Congress of Music Therapy, Washington, 33–9.

Lord, C., Rutter, M., Goode, S., Heemsberger, J., Jordan, H., Manwhood, L. and Schopler, E. (1989) 'Autistic Diagnostic Observation Schedule: A Standardised Observation of Communicative and Social Behaviour.' *Journal of Autism and Developmental Disorders 19*, 2, 185–212.

Molyneux, C. (2001) 'Short-term Music Therapy within a Child and Adolescent Mental Health Service: Description of a Developing Service.' MA thesis, Anglia Ruskin University.

Nocker-Ribaupierre, M. (1999) 'Premature Birth and Music Therapy.' In T. Wigram and de J. Backer (eds) *Clinical Applications of Music Therapy in Developmental Disability, Paediatrics and Neurology.* London: Jessica Kingsley Publishers, 47–65.

Nordoff, P. and Robbins, C. (1971) *Therapy in Music for Handicapped Children.* London: Victor Gollancz.

Nordoff, P. amd Robbins, C. (1977) *Creative Music Therapy.* New York: John Day Co.

Oldfield, A. (1992) 'Teaching Music Therapy Students on Clinical Placements: Some Observations.' *Journal of British Music Therapy 6*, 1, 13–17.

Oldfield, A. (1993a) 'A Study of the Way Music Therapists Analyse their Work.' *Journal of British Music Therapy 7*, 1, 14–22.

Oldfield, A. (1993b) 'Music Therapy with Families.' In M. Heal and T. Wigram (eds) *Music Therapy in Health and Education.* London: Jessica Kingsley Publishers, 46–54.

Oldfield, A. (2000) 'Music Therapy as a Contribution to the Diagnosis made by the Staff Team in Child and Family Psychiatry: An Initial Description of a Methodology that is Still Emerging through Clinical Practice.' In T. Wigram (ed) *Assessment and Evaluation in the Arts Therapies.* St Albans: Harper House Publications, 93–101.

Oldfield, A. (2004) 'Music Therapy with Children on the Autistic Spectrum: Approaches Derived from Clinical Practice and Research.' PhD thesis, available from Anglia Ruskin University.

Oldfield, A. (2006) *Interactive Music Therapy: A Positive Approach: Music Therapy at a Child Development Centre.* London: Jessica Kingsley Publishers.

Oldfield, A. and Adams, M. (1990) 'The Effects of Music Therapy on a Group of Profoundly Handicapped Adults.' *Journal of Mental Deficiency Research 34*, 107–25.

Oldfield, A. and Bunce, L. (2001) 'Mummy Can Play Too: Short-term Music Therapy with Mothers and Young Children.' *British Journal of Music Therapy 15*, 27–36.

Oldfield, A. and Cramp, R. (1992) 'Music Therapy at the Child Development Centre, Cambridge.' Training video produced by Anglia Ruskin University, available from the British Society for Music Therapy.

Oldfield, A. and Cramp, R. (1994) 'Timothy: Music Therapy with a Little Boy who has Asperger Syndrome.' Training video produced by Anglia Ruskin University, available from the British Society for Music Therapy.

Oldfield, A. and Franke, C. (2005) 'Improvised Songs and Stories in Music Therapy Diagnostic Assessments at a Unit for Child and Family Psychiatry: A Music Therapist's and a Psychotherapist's Perspective.' In F. Baker and T. Wigram (eds) *Song Writing, Methods, Techniques and Clinical Applications for Music Therapy Clinicians, Educators and Students.* London: Jessica Kingsley Publishers.

Oldfield, A. and Nudds, J. (2002) 'Joshua and Barry: Music Therapy with a Partially Sighted Little Boy with Cerebral Palsy.' Training video produced by Anglia Ruskin University, available from the British Society for Music Therapy.

Oldfield, A. and Nudds, J. (2005) 'The Croft: A Unit for Child and Family Psychiatry in Cambridge.' Training video produced by Anglia Ruskin University, available from the British Society for Music Therapy.

Oldfield, A., Bunce, L. and Adams, M. (2003) 'An Investigation into Short-term Music Therapy with Mothers and Young Children.' *British Journal of Music Therapy 17*, 1, 26–45.

Oldfield, A., MacDonald, R. and Nudds, J. (1999) 'Training as a Music Therapist: The MA in Music Therapy at APU.' Training video produced by Anglia Ruskin University, available from the British Society for Music Therapy.

Oldfield, A., MacDonald, R. and Nudds, J. (2000) 'Music Therapy for Children on the Autistic Spectrum.' Training video produced by Anglia Ruskin University, available from the British Society for Music Therapy.

Rogers, P. (1992) 'Issues in Working with Sexually Abused Clients in Music Therapy.' *Journal of British Music Therapy 6*, 2, 5–15.

Rogers, P. (2000) 'Truth or Illusion: Evidence-based Practice in the Real World.' In J. Robarts (ed) *Music Therapy Research: Growing Perspectives in Theory and Practice.* London: BSMT Publications, 11–33.

Saperston, M.S. (1999) 'The Relationship of Cognitive Language, Melodic Development of Normal Children, Children with Developmental Delays, and Adults with Mental Retardation.' In B. Wilson and E. York (co-chairs) *Proceedings of the Institute on Music Therapy Assessment*, World Congress of Music Therapy, Washington, 21–6.

Siegel, B., Anders, T., Ciaranello, R., Beinenstock, B. and Kraemer, H. (1986) 'Empirically Derived Classification of the Autistic Syndrome.' *Journal of Autism and Developmental Disorders, 18,* 81–98.

Siegel, S. (1956) *Non-parametric Statistics.* Toronto: McGraw-Hill.

Stern, D. (1985) *The Interpersonal World of the Infant.* New York: Basic Books.

Stern, D. (1995) *The Motherhood Constellation: A Unified View of Parent–Infant Psychotherapy.* New York: Basic Books.

Stern, D. (1996) 'The Temporal Structure of Interactions between Parents and Infants: The Earliest Music?' Unpublished paper presented at the 8th Congress of Music Therapy, 'Sound and Psyche', Hamburg, Germany.

Stige, B. (2002) *Culture Centred Music Therapy.* Phoenixville, PA: Barcelona Publishers.

Trevarthen, C., Aitken, K., Papoudi, D. and Robarts, J. (1996) *Children with Autism: Diagnosis and Intervention to Meet their Needs.* London: Jessica Kingsley Publishers.

Tyler, H. (2001) 'Group music therapy with children and adolescents.' Paper presented at the 5th European Music Therapy Congress, Naples, Italy and at the British Society for Music Therapy.

Warwick, A. (1988) 'Questions and Reflections on Research.' *Journal of British Music Therapy 2,* 2, 5–8.

Warwick, A. (1995) 'Music Therapy in the Education Service: Research with Autistic Children.' In T. Wigram, B. Saperston and R. West (eds) *The Art and Science of Music Therapy: A Handbook.* Chur, Switzerland: Harwood Academic Publishers, 209–25.

Wells, N. (1988) 'An Individual Music Therapy Assessment Procedure for Emotionally Disturbed Young Adolescents.' *Arts in Psychotherapy 15,* 47–54.

Wheeler, B. (1995) 'Introduction: Overview of Music Therapy Research.' In B. Wheeler (ed) *Music Therapy Research: Quantitative and Qualitative Perspectives.* Phoenixville: Barcelona Publishers, 3–15.

Wigram, T. (1995) 'A Model of Assessment and Differential Diagnoses of Handicap in Children through the Medium of Music Therapy.' In T. Wigram, B. Saperston and R. West (eds) *The Art and Science of Music Therapy: A Handbook.* Chur, Switzerland: Harwood Academic Publishers, 181–93.

Wigram, T. (1999) 'Contact in Music: Analysis of Musical Behaviours in Children with Communication Disorders and Pervasive Developmental Disorders for Differential Diagnoses.' In T. Wigram and J. de Backer (eds) *Clinical Applications of Music Therapy in Developmental Disability, Paediatrics and Neurology.* London: Jessica Kingsley Publishers, 69–93.

Wigram, T. (2000) 'A Model of Diagnostic Assessment and Analysis of Musical Data in Music Therapy.' In T. Wigram (ed) *Assessment and Evaluation in the Arts Therapies.* St Albans: Harper House Publications, 77–92.

Wigram, T. (2002) 'Indications in Music Therapy: Evidence from Assessment that can Identify the Expectations of Music Therapy as a Treatment for Autistic Spectrum Disorder (ASD). Meeting the Challenge of Evidence-based Practice.' *British Journal of Music Therapy 16,* 1, 11–28.

Winnicott, D. (1960) *Playing and Reality.* UK: Pelican Publications.

Winnicott, D. (1971) *Holding and Interpretation.* New York: Grove Press.

York, E. (1999) 'A Test–Retest Reliability Study of the Residual Music Skills Test Assessment.' In B. Wilson and E. York (co-chairs) *Proceedings of the Institute on Music Therapy Assessment,* World Congress of Music Therapy, Washington, 43–7.

Subject Index

Author Index